The
ROENTGENOGRAPHIC DIAGNOSIS
of
RENAL MASS LESIONS

A Monograph in

MODERN CONCEPTS OF RADIOLOGY
NUCLEAR MEDICINE AND ULTRASOUND

Series Editor

LEWIS E. ETTER, M.D., F.A.C.R.

Professor of Radiology
Western Psychiatric Institute
and Falk Clinic
Presbyterian-University Hospital
School of Medicine
University of Pittsburgh
Pittsburgh, Pennsylvania

The
ROENTGENOGRAPHIC
DIAGNOSIS
of
RENAL MASS LESIONS

By

ERICH K. LANG, M.D.

Professor and Chairman
Department of Radiology
Louisiana State University Medical Center
School of Medicine in Shreveport
Shreveport, Louisiana

WARREN H. GREEN, INC.

St. Louis, Missouri, U.S.A.

Published by
WARREN H. GREEN, INC.
10 South Brentwood Blvd.
St. Louis, Missouri 63105, U.S.A.

Library of Congress Catalog Card No. 70-125008

Printed in the United States of America
4–A   (175)

FOREWORD

R OENTGEN DIAGNOSIS IN ALL FIELDS, but particularly in urology, has been undergoing an unheralded but nonetheless extremely significant metamorphosis. Hitherto, the scope of roentgen diagnostic evaluation of the urinary excretory system was limited to the investigation of normal and morbid anatomy. In the recent past, however, the demand for a final and definitive diagnosis has been established for both clinical and laboratory diagnostic examinations. This change of diagnostic goal and concept has prompted diagnostic radiology to acquire a new dimension.

The mere roentgen diagnosis of "space-occupying lesions of the kidney" is no longer acceptable and a differentiation of inflammatory, benign and malignant neoplastic lesions involving the kidneys is expected from the radiologist today.

With this demand in mind, diagnostic radiology has been expanded by innumerable special roentgenographic techniques and the data presentation has been advanced by the introduction of technically advanced equipment.

It is hoped that this monograph will bring together the vast amount of previously scattered information on newer and special roentgenographic techniques designed for assessment and differentiation of renal mass lesions and that it will meet the need for a comprehensive and authoritative survey on these diagnostic roentgenographic examinations. The presentation will not only attempt to establish a rationale for proper sequence in which a special examination modality should be deployed but also acquaint the reader with the diagnostic accuracy which can be expected each and every one of these examinations.

No book ever reaches fruition as a result of the author's efforts alone. The efforts of my secretary, Mrs. Kathryn Wendt, and Mr. Gordon Maxcy of the Art and Photography Department at Confederate Memorial Medical Center are acknowledged with sincere thanks.

ERICH   K.   LANG, M.D.

CONTENTS

TABLES

viii

The

ROENTGENOGRAPHIC DIAGNOSIS

of

RENAL MASS LESIONS

CHAPTER I

INTRODUCTION

THE LAST DECADE has witnessed a change in the diagnostic goal of the assessment of renal mass lesions (21, 101). In the past, the obligation of the diagnostician ceased after establishing the diagnosis of a space-occupying lesion in the kidney. Today, differentiation of the various types of space-occupying lesions is considered mandatory (75, 76, 121, 123). The need for the development of various diagnostic tests capable of differentiating and assessing renal cysts and tumors was established by a change of the predominant age group in whom asymptomatic space-occupying lesions were first recognized and by the demand to establish a definitive diagnosis to obviate surgical exploration (144).

The change in statistical occurrence of cyst and tumor is, undoubtedly, related to the marked increase in the use of intravenous urography as a routine screening examination in a urologic patient group which shows a rapid preponderance of patients past the fifth decade. Prior to 1926, not a single case of renal cyst was found among 12,500 admissions to the Brady Urologic Institute, Johns Hopkins Hospital. In the 1940's, the incidence rate of cysts was considered one-half that of carcinoma. Today, however, the incidence rate of cysts presenting as symptomatic and asymptomatic space-occupying lesions exceeds, by far, that of tumors. This, undoubtedly, reflects our increased ability to recognize space-occupying lesions and the expanded use of screening intravenous urography in a urologic patient population that has substantially increased in average age. Renal carcinoma is not a common malignancy; it constitutes no more than 1 to 2 percent of all cancers (242). Renal cysts, however, are found in 3 to 5 percent of all routine autopsies (41). Our ability to recognize such space-occupying lesions is best denoted by reports in the recent literature claiming a 2 percent incidence of renal mass deformity seen on the routine intravenous urograms performed on patients requiring prostatectomy (33).

Our recently gained ability to recognize many asymptomatic space-occupying lesions that evaded detection in the past necessitates a reevaluation of our concepts of management of such lesions (101, 145). In the past, the demonstration of a space-occupying lesion in the kidney almost certainly indicated the presence of a neoplasm. Hence, surgical exploration was the method of choice. Today, the diagnosis of an asymptomatic space-occupying lesion in the kidney would more often indicate the presence of a cyst than a tumor. In the past, many authorities have advocated exploration of all asymptomatic space-occupying lesions in all patients without medical contraindication to surgery. This concept must be reevaluated in the light of the statistical data of curability of a given mass lesion against the incidence of surgical mortality and morbidity for the patient (114, 144, 146, 223, 236, 237).

The incidence of surgical mortality and morbidity accelerates sharply with rising age and casts considerable doubt on the efficacy of exploration as a diagnostic procedure (144). Lassen analyzed the progressive increase of operative mortality rate in all elective procedures for various age groups (168.) An operative mortality rate of 2 percent was established for the 40-year age group. For the 65-year age group this rose to almost 10 percent and for the 80-year age group, the unacceptable figure of over 25 percent had been reached. The increased mortality or permanent disability in this older age group was confirmed by Plaine, *et al.,* who reported a mortality-morbidity incidence rate of 2.4 percent in their patients operated for serous cysts (223). Moreover, 11 percent of unnecessary nephrectomies resulted from exploration of space-occupying lesions either because the benign nature of the lesion could not be determined at operation or because hemorrhage had been impossible to control otherwise. Apart from the significant risk of surgical exploration, this procedure is not infallible in the detection of cancer and cases of surgically missed neoplasms have been reported (101, 116).

In order to ascertain the statistical significance of these deliberations, Plaine established the formula "chance of missing carcinoma = incidence of cancer × percent inaccuracy of tests" (Table I). The diagnostic accuracy, therefore, depends on appropriate assignment of the patient to a group with an established

TABLE I*
CHANCE OF MISSING CANCER = INCIDENCE OF CANCER ×
ACCURACY OF TEST

Groups with Known Incidence of Carcinoma	Chance of Missing Carcinoma by Arteriography or Nephrotomography (90% Accuracy)
All carcinoma	10%
50% of all carcinoma (symptomatic and/or with stigmata of malignancy)	5%
5% of all carcinoma (asymptomatic without stigmata of malignancy)	0.5%

*Adapted from: Plaine, L. I., and Hinman, Frank, Jr.: Malignancy in asymptomatic renal masses. J Urol 94:342-347, 1965.

statistical incidence of cancer and on available statistical data on the percentage accuracy of the composite tests deployed for ascertaining this diagnosis (223). After eliminating all patients with symptoms or other stigmata of renal malignancy, a group of only 79 patients out of 387 remained in Plaine's series of renal mass lesions (223). Of these remaining 79 patients, only 4 were found to have a malignancy. Plaine argues, on the basis of statistical deliberations, that only 1 carcinoma in 220 patients with renal mass lesions would be missed in the subgroup without symptoms or stigmata of malignancy and without nephrotomographically or angiographically identifiable neoplasm. The incidence rate of death or permanent disability resulting from exploratory surgery in this group of patients, however, approximates 2.4 percent. He, therefore, advocates reliance on laboratory and x-ray evaluation of malignancy since the actual probability of finding a carcinoma and curing it is only 0.25 percent whereas the chance of death or permanent disability from an operative intervention is 2.4 percent (223).

The paramount importance of early diagnosis of renal cell carcinoma and the use of radical procedures adapted to the stage of

the neoplasm have been emphasized in the recent surgical literature (145, 146, 233, 236, 237). The significance of the clinical
stage of a renal carcinoma in respect to the curability of the lesion
was first pointed out by Kaufman and Mims (146) (Table II).

TABLE II*

SURVIVAL CURVES ACCORDING TO DEGREE OF INVASION AND
BASED ON 100 OF OUR CASES. (FROM KAUFMAN AND MIMS)

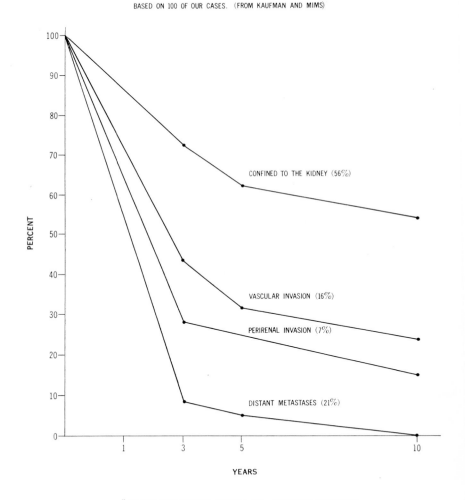

*ADAPTED FROM: KAUFMAN, JOSEPH J., M.D.: REASONS FOR NEPHRECTOMY.
PALLIATIVE AND CURATIVE.   JAMA 204: 145-146, 1968.

In their series of 100 patients, a greater than 50 percent 10-year survival rate is noted in those with lesions confined to the kidney, accounting for 56 percent of the total group. In patients demonstrating renal vein invasion, 16 percent of the total series, the 10-year survival drops to 25 percent. In the presence of perirenal extension of disease, the 10-year survival is reduced to less than 20 percent. However, if distant metastases were present at the time of diagnosis, a finding occurring in 21 percent of the total series, there were no 10-year survivors (Table II).

The importance of early diagnosis of renal cell carcinoma to guarantee early and adequate surgical treatment is self-evident from this tabulation (Tables II and III). The pathologic grade of

TABLE III*
5 YEAR SURVIVAL OF PATIENTS WITH HYPERNEPHROMA OF VARIOUS STAGE IRREGARDLESS OF TREATMENT

Arteriographic Stage	Total No.	5 Year Survival	% 5 yr. Survival	Lost for Follow up
I	15	9	60%	2
II-a	12	6	50%	2
b	4	1	25%	1
c	9	1	11%	2
III-a	9	1	11%	2
b	2	0	0	1
c	1	0	0	0
d	8	1	12.5%	2
	60	19	31.6	12

*Courtesy, Lang, E.K.—Radiology.

the tumor and cell type, likewise, influence the survival figures by the propensity of undifferentiated lesions to cause early local invasion and early distant metastases (12, 145). Radical nephrectomy with retroperitoneal lymph adenectomy appears to offer a better prognosis than a conservative surgical approach particularly in patients with renal vein involvement, perirenal extension, or local lymphatic involvement (24). Robson reported a 10 year survival rate of 63.3 percent in patients subjected to a radical nephrectomy versus 22 percent in a large collected series treated by simple nephrectomy (237). The value of renal arteriography for assessment of extension of the tumor into the perirenal area, involvement of the renal vein, and demonstration of distal metastatic implants has been emphasized by many authors (1, 3, 5, 7, 18, 23, 38, 75, 78, 80, 141, 142, 143, 144, 161, 162, 163, 165, 184, 193, 205, 210, 228, 234, 237, 248, 276).

The last but probably most important single factor influencing diagnostic goals is the sum total accuracy of diagnostic procedures deployed for definitive assessment of such lesions.

Differentiation of cyst from tumor on basis of clinical criteria is difficult if not impossible (16, 96). It has been emphasized that painless hematuria is highly suggestive of renal cell carcinoma. However, in most series hematuria is found in only 50 to 60 percent of the patients with renal cell carcinoma (133, 211). Gregg, in his series, found hematuria in 50 percent of the patients with renal cell carcinoma and in 33 percent of those with cysts (115). Pain was as common in his patients with cysts as in those with tumor. A palpable mass, however, was more frequent in cysts. Hypertension, again, was present with the same frequency in both conditions (133, 153). The classical triad of renal mass, pain, and hematuria is usually found in less than 25 percent of the cases (122).

Anemia and an elevated erythrocyte sedimentation rate are definitely more frequent in tumors, nevertheless, intercurrent disease entities may occasion a similar pattern in patients with renal cysts (114). Elevated urinary beta glucuronidase levels, likewise, favor the diagnosis of a hypernephroma (246). However, similar elevation of enzyme levels may be caused by active pyelonephritis. Elevation of C-reactive protein is a finding of such nonspecific nature that one should caution against utilizing this data for differentiation of renal tumors and cysts.

The relative infrequency of calcifications in tumors demonstrable on plain roentgenograms mitigates against successful use of this criterion. Moreover, the presence of calcifications in proven renal cell carcinoma has been reported as lower than 2 percent and as high as 35 percent whereas that of renal cysts is generally considered to be in the 3 percent range; findings which emphasize the definite overlap of this criterion in a substantial percentage of cysts and tumors (122, 165, 248) (Table IV). Even the demonstration of crescent-shaped calcifications carries no particular diag-

TABLE IV*

INCIDENCE OF CALCIFICATION IN 225 RENAL MASS LESIONS

Type of Mass Lesion	No. of Cases	No. Calcified
Simple cysts	72	2 (3%)
Polycystic disease	17	1 (6%)
Renal-cell carcinoma	66	9 (14%)
Metastatic carcinoma	37	0
Wilms's tumor	13	1 (8%)
Neuroblastoma	15	8 (53%)
Renal sarcoma	1	1
Renal pelvic carcinoma	1	1
Renal adenoma	1	1
Renal artery aneurysm	1	1
Adrenal cyst	1	1

*Adapted from: Phillips, T. L., M.D., *et al.*: Calcification in renal masses: An eleven-year survey. Radiology 80:786-794, 1963.

nostic significance and may be seen both in cysts and tumors (252). In general, however, it can be stated that the incidence rate of calcifications is higher in renal cell carcinoma than in simple cysts (221) (Table IV).

Calyceal disturbances seen on the intravenous pyelogram may result from cysts as well as tumors (42). Elongation of the calyces and infundibula is more commonly found in neoplasms. Displacement and separation of calyces and splaying of infundibula may be seen in both cysts and neoplasms. Compression of calyces, again, is encountered in both cysts and neoplasms. Amputation of calyces or irregular invasion of calyces or infundibula, however, is highly suggestive of neoplasms. Nonetheless, invasion of the pyelocalyceal system and amputation of calyces may occasionally occur with cysts. A definitive diagnosis is, therefore, rarely possible on basis of the intravenous or retrograde pyelogram. Besides, it has been proven conclusively on roentgenograms of postmortem specimen that lesions up to 2 cm in diameter cannot be identified with confidence on the intravenous urogram (58).

The necessity for higher detail demonstration of renal mass lesions prompted Evans to introduce nephrotomography (87). Particularly in conjunction with the intravenous drip infusion technique of contrast media, nephrotomography provides a simple and relatively reliable modality for assessment of renal mass lesions (62, 247). An accuracy rate of 95 percent has been claimed for this technique (87, 88, 89, 90) (Table V). However, it should be emphasized that this accuracy rate can only be achieved in those cases demonstrating characteristic nephrotomographic features (37, 218). Since almost one-half of all patients present with equivocal nephrotomographic findings, the overall accuracy is usually reduced to approximately 75 percent (37, 218). None-the-less the usefulness of this technique for assessment of necrotic lesions and particularly of small lesions has been stressed (37, 85, 126).

TABLE V**
ACCURACY OF NEPHROTOMOGRAPHY*

Diagnosis	No. of Patients	Accuracy	
		Correct	Incorrect
Cyst	147	145	2 carcinomas
Neoplasm	38	34	4 cysts
Indeterminate	14	0	9 cysts and 5 carcinomas

*From Witten *et al.*
**Adapted from Evans, John, M.D.: The accuracy of diagnostic radiology. JAMA: 131-134, 1968.

Radioisotope scanning techniques first utilized mercury 203 chlormerodrin. Both cysts and tumors presented as a negative defect and differentiation necessitated computation of count rate ratios over both kidneys (30, 127, 202). This method proved highly unreliable and complicated for differentiation of renal cysts and tumors. However, rapid gamma ray scintillation camera scanning after intravenous injection of technetium 99 M pertechnetate as suggested by Rosenthal provides a technique capable of recognizing abnormal tumor vascularity and, hence, differentiating tumors from cysts or areas of ischemia (240). In spite of encouraging early reports, large statistics will have to be compiled before definitive credibility can be accorded to this examination technique.

Arteriography is, undoubtedly, one of the most reliable examination techniques for differentiation of various renal mass lesions (5, 34). Overzealous interpretation of questionable findings and substandard studies have undermined the reputation of this modality in the past (270, 276). The erroneous conclusion that lack of proper visualization of the renal vein on late phase arteriograms indicates the presence of tumor invasion of the renal vein is one of the outstanding examples of illogical and unsupported diagnostic reasoning (276). Watson *et al.*, for example, reported that in their series of 100 patients with renal cell carcinoma, the renal vein failed to visualize in 52 instances. However, only 11 of these patients showed evidence of tumor invasion into the renal vein on gross or microscopic examination. Lack of proper visualization of the renal vein is more often a function of inappropriate or inadequate injection of a contrast medium bolus into the artery than of primary obstruction or invasion of the renal vein (276). The same authors caution against undue reliance on the observation of opacification of collateral veins as an indicator for renal vein thrombosis. In at least two of their patients, exploration failed to verify the presence of any significant renal vein abnormality in spite of arteriographic demonstration of substantial collateral vein opacification (276). However, in another 14 patients, Watson was able to confirm the diagnosis of renal vein invasion by tumor suggested on arteriogram on basis of filling defects in the main renal vein or redirection of venous drainage via dilated collateral veins.

The possibility of simultaneous occurrence of renal cyst and tumor has been cited as the main objection to relying on diagnostic modalities short of operative exploration for establishing the diagnosis of a renal mass lesion. The reported incidence rate of such lesions varies from 0 to 30 percent (144, 281). It is suspected that concurrent malignant tumor has often been missed after the diagnosis of renal cyst had been established and that the actual rate of coexistence of cyst and tumor is as high as $2\frac{1}{2}$ percent (42, 60, 110, 164, 171, 228, 231). It is postulated that reported higher incidence rates of such concurrent tumor and cyst are primarily due to inclusion of cystic degenerating renal cell carcinoma and cyst adenoma in this group of patients. While cystic or necrotic tumors should be identifiable on basis of thick and irregular walls seen on nephrotomography, tumors projecting into a cyst or arising in the cyst wall are rarely demonstrable by this technique (37). Selective renal angiography, particularly if enhanced by preceding injection of adrenalin hydrochloride, has been found reliable for identification of abnormal vessels not only in cystic tumors but also in small tumors causing a distal cyst and in tumors arising from the cyst wall (3, 130, 140, 141, 228).

Cyst puncture with aspiration of contents, histochemical and histopathological examination of the aspirant, and double contrast study coupled with laminography has been found extremely dependable in the identification of coexistent cysts and tumors (23, 63, 67, 69, 77, 108, 144, 154, 157, 158, 164, 176, 177, 186, 216, 221, 285, 286). The observation of bloody or discolored fluid, and increased fat content on histochemical examination of the aspirant along with roentgenographic identification of tumors in cysts has been found reliable for the diagnosis of coexistent cyst and tumor. Double contrast study, aided by tomography, is capable of identifying irregular contour margins or masses protruding into the lumen of the cyst. Superimposition of the opacified cyst on the negative filling defect seen on the nephrotomogram ascertains whether the entire mass lesion is adequately explained by the opacified cyst. An existing disparity between the opacified cyst and the suggested mass lesion on the nephrotomogram should be resolved by further puncture and aspiration attempts designed to delineate other cystic masses or to establish the presence of a solid tumor mass.

The sum total of today's available roentgenographic techniques including infusion pyelography, infusion nephrotomography, selective renal angiography aided by adrenalin injection, and cyst puncture, aspiration, histochemical and histopathologic examination of the aspirant, and double contrast study of the cyst probably not only equals but betters the diagnostic accuracy obtained by surgical exploration of renal mass lesions (116). Reliance on these techniques is advocated to spare the patient unnecessary exploration with the resultant morbidity and mortality and to furnish the surgeon reliable preoperative evaluation and staging of a malignant mass lesion (165, 193, 276). The appropriate and widespread use of the entire gamut of diagnostic techniques for the assessment of renal mass lesions will not only furnish an accurate preoperative diagnosis and avoid many an unnecessary exploration with the resulting morbidity and late sequelae but will, even more importantly, furnish definitive data for accurate staging of malignant lesions and, hence, permit a more individualized and radical therapeutic approach (145, 146, 162, 163, 165, 193, 236,237) .

CHAPTER II

RENAL TUMORS

R ENAL TUMORS ARE, numerically, only a small component in the total group of urologic disorders but are in the foreground of diagnostic concern because of their propensity to mimic other urologic conditions. The fact that more than two-thirds of all tumors arising from the kidney are adenocarcinomas (hypernephroma) emphasizes the impact and consequence of the diagnosis of a renal neoplasm (184). In its statistical perspective to other neoplasms, renal cell carcinoma is relegated to the position of a relatively rare malignancy constituting less than 2 percent of all cancers (242). The pathophysiology of this neoplasm and particularly the tumor-immune mechanism that was first studied in patients with hypernephroma has lifted this neoplasm from its numerical position of frequency of occurrence and assigned it special key position in the field of investigation of tumor-immune mechanisms and host suppression of tumors (242).

Tumors of the kidney can be divided into two large groups: 1) those arising from the parenchyma, and 2) those arising from the renal pelvis and calyces. To simplify further discussion and to serve as reference, a simple classification encompassing all renal tumors is outlined:

    I. Parenchymal renal tumors
       A. Benign parenchymal renal tumors
          1. Epithelial tumors
             a. Adenomas (papillary, alveolar, and tubular types)
          2. Mesenchymal tumors
             a. Fibromas
             b. Myomas
             c. Lipomas

        d. Angiomas

        e. Mixed tumors (hamartomas)

        f. Myxomas

  B. Malignant parenchymal tumors

    1. Epithelial tumors

        a. Adenocarcinoma (clear-cell carcinoma, hypernephroma)

    2. Mesenchymal tumors

        a. Sarcomas

    3. Embryonal tumors

        a. Wilms' tumors

        b. Embryonal adenosarcomas

    4. Tumors involving the cortex secondarily

II. Tumors of the renal pelvis and ureter

  A. Benign tumors

    1. Epithelial (benign papillomas)

    2. Nonepithelial

        a. Fibromas

        b. Myomas

        c. Myxomas

  B. Malignant tumors

    1. Epithelial tumors (transitional cell epitheliomas, squamous cell carcinomas)

    2. Adenocarcinomas

    3. Nonepithelial (mesenchymal tumors, sarcomas)

HYPERNEPHROMAS

The axiom that locally invasive and metastatic cancers run an inexorable course is met with many exceptions in renal cell carcinoma (145). The well known fact that regression of metastases may occur following nephrectomy and removal of the primary lesion is one of the outstanding individualistic behavior patterns of renal cell carcinoma (9, 12, 17, 18, 92, 162, 233, 242). A possible explanation for this mechanism has been proposed; immunologic paralysis due to the overwhelming number of cancer cells may be overcome by removing the bulk of the tumor. Immunologic tolerance is then converted to immunologic competence by freeing resources of the host defense mechanism to attack the metastases (242). This concept of tumor-immune mechanism in conjunction with impressive survival statistics following radical nephrectomy tend to place increasing emphasis on surgical approach to this problem (145, 146, 233, 236, 237). Increasing evidence of curability of certain stages and grades of renal cell carcinoma by radical nephrectomy and lymph node dissection possibly combined with radiation therapy or chemotherapy emphasizes the necessity for accurate preoperative assessment of these lesions (95, 99, 114, 145, 146, 162, 165, 219, 236, 237). A definitive evaluation of the virtues of certain surgical procedures versus other procedures has to be based on an assessment of cure rate of accurately staged and graded renal lesions to permit a valid comparison (Tables II and III). Robson reported a 60 percent 10-year survival of renal cell carcinoma if confined to the kidney at the time of radical nephrectomy (237). The 10-year survival dropped to 37 percent if renal vein invasion or lymphatic invasion was present. If, however, distant metastases were present, there were no 10-year survivors. This statistic is well supported by a report by Kaufman who showed a 10-year survival of better than 50 percent in patients with carcinoma confined to the kidney at the time of removal by nephrectomy. In the presence of vascular invasion, only 25 percent were alive at 10 years. If perirenal extension was treated surgically, 14 percent were alive at 10 years. In the presence of distant metastases, there were no 10-year survivors (Table II) (24, 145).

The paramount importance of classification and staging of renal cell carcinoma is apparent when perusing the statistics (Tables II and III). Adaptation of treatment modalities to the stage of the disease will, undoubtedly, result in better survival for each respective stage. Whether this is by more extensive and radical surgical resection as proposed by Robson or whether this can be achieved by nephrectomy combined with pre- or postoperative irradiation or chemotherapy as advocated by Riches and Flocks can be determined only by compilation of data from large series painstakingly assessed preoperatively and properly staged to permit a valid comparison (99, 233, 236,237). A comparison of the effectiveness of various techniques based on survival statistics derived from unstaged and unclassified renal cell carcinoma serves no useful scientific purpose because of the marked disparity of the types of lesions prevalent in different series. Robson, for example, found in his series 38 percent of renal cell carcinoma confined to the kidney, 17 percent extending into the perirenal fat, 31 percent with vascular or lymphatic invasion, and 14 percent with distant metastases (237). Kaufman and Mims had 56 percent of the lesions confined to the kidney in their series, 16 percent with vascular invasion, 7 percent with perirenal invasion, and 21 percent with distant metastases (146). McDonald and Priestley noted tumor thrombosis of the renal vein in 54 percent of their cases (184). The inferior vena cava was involved in 9 percent of the patients in Everson's series (92). Stackpole reported extension of tumor through the renal capsule in 72 percent of his patients (258). Regional lymph node involvement varied from 5 to 38 percent in various series. In some autopsy series, pulmonary metastases were recorded as high as 55.9 percent (114). On basis of this gross disparity of the type of lesion found in the patient material of various investigators, a comparative study of the effectiveness of certain techniques can be carried out only if the stage of the disease is established in a uniform manner.

The clinical criteria alerting the physician to the possible presence of a hypernephroma are of little or no value for the staging of this disease (116, 133, 211). The triad of "hematuria, pain, and mass" has been emphasized as a diagnostic feature. Its occurrence has been reported as high as 90 percent and as low as 15 percent by various investigators. It should be emphasized, however, that these criteria are in no way diagnostic of the presence of a renal cell carcinoma. Hoffman reported hematuria in 50 percent of patients with carcinoma and in 33 percent of those with cysts (133). Pain was as frequent in his cases with cysts as in those with tumor. A palpable mass was more frequent in cysts. Hypertension was present with the same frequency in both conditions. Ochsner found hematuria in 60 percent of his patients with renal cell carcinoma, pain in 40 percent, a palpable mass in 38 percent, fever in 25 percent and the triad of "hematuria, pain, and renal mass" in only 15 percent of the patients (211). Apart from the somewhat overemphasized "surgical triad," pyrexia, polycytemia, hypocalcemia, hypertension, leukemoid reaction, salt-losing syndrome, left heart failure secondary to arteriovenous fistulae, anemia and Cushing's syndrome have been reported as medical syndromes occurring in patients with hypernephromas (1, 107). While some of these observations infer certain clinical complications, such as pyrexia suggesting the presence of necrosis in the tumor, left heart failure suggesting an arteriovenous fistula, palpable metastases ascertaining metastatic disease, the sum total knowledge of the stage and condition of the tumor is not significantly enhanced by these criteria (11, 12).

Laboratory findings such as elevation of the erythrocyte sedimentation rate, elevation of the urinary beta glucuronidase levels, and anemia are frequently encountered in patients with hypernephroma (114, 246). While these data are useful for differentiation of benign versus malignant renal mass lesions, they do not necessarily permit conclusions as to the extent of the involvement by neoplasm.

Plain roentgenograms of the abdomen may sometimes suggest the presence of a tumor involving the renal cortex on basis of a cortical irregularity and unilateral enlargement (Fig. 1a, b). In cases of very large tumors, the normal renal outline may have been replaced by a huge soft tissue mass presenting in the region of the kidney (84, 100). Scattered and mottled calcifications likewise may denote the presence of a renal tumor. The incidence of calcifications in known renal carcinoma has been reported with marked disparity; reports range in incidence rate from less than 2 to 35 percent (164, 222, 248, 276). Most authors concur that scattered and mottled calcifications are more common in renal tumors than in cysts or benign tumors. Phillips reported calcifications in 14 percent in renal carcinomas and in only 3 percent in simple cysts; however, this figure rose to 6 percent in polycystic disease (222). Spherical or shell-like calcifications are more frequently seen in renal cysts, nevertheless, the diagnosis of a renal tumor cannot be excluded on basis of this observation (47, 243, 252) (Fig. 24, 25). Shockman reported ring-shaped renal calcifications in two renal carcinomas and in two cysts (252). Even the concurrence of calcifications in a renal carcinoma and in a cyst in the same kidney has been reported (152). The presence of calcification in a tumor is usually considered a grave prognostic sign (122, 211, 248). Schreiber found that calcifications in renal tumor increased the likelihood of unresectability from 21 to 29 percent in his series of 63 renal cell carcinomas (248).

On the intravenous urogram the tumor may be reflected by overall enlargement of the involved kidney or irregularity of the kidney outline particularly if the tumor enlarges toward the periphery (Fig. 1). Displacement of the infundibula and calyces may likewise result. Elongation of the calyces is the most pathognomonic deformity seen in cortical tumors. However, elongation of the calyces may also occur in the normal kidney and may be seen with benign space-occupying lesions. The only reliable criterion for differentiation is demonstration of an abnormal termination of the elongated calyx, partial or complete obliteration or direct destruction by an invasive tumor (Fig. 2) (57, 59). A bulbous appearance of the calyx may result if a tumor is compressing or invading the infundibulum (Fig. 47a). The extent or number of calyces involved by such a process do not necessarily reflect the invasiveness or size of the tumor. In diffuse infiltrating tumors, the calyces have been stretched to unusual length producing a bizarre appearance on the intravenous urogram which has been described by the term "spider leg" deformity (59). In large and advanced renal cell carcinomas, only a portion of the calyces may be visualized resulting in a picture of detached deposits of contrast medium reflecting extensive destruction of the calyces and opacification of the remaining functioning components. In general, calyceal deformities can be demonstrated by both intravenous urogram and, particularly, by infusion pyelograms as well as by retrograde pyelograms (Fig. 3). Only in rare instances will the tumor occlude distal portions of the calyx preventing introduction of contrast material via the retrograde route.

Not infrequently, tumors encroach on the pelvis occasioning

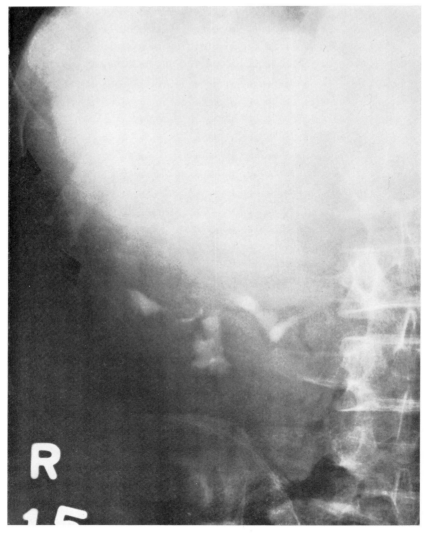

FIGURE 1a, 1b. The upper pole of the right kidney shows irregular enlargement. The magnitude of the enlargement, however, is best appreciated on the retroperitoneal gas study.

flattening, elongation, narrowing, irregular filling defects, and deformity of the pelvis, but cause only rarely occlusion of the ure-

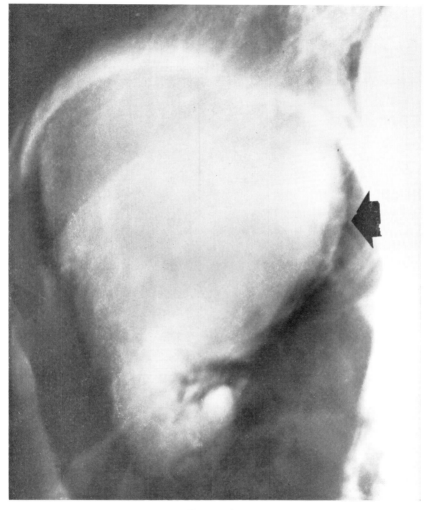

FIGURE 1b.

teropelvic junction (59). The displaced and abnormal position of the renal pelvis may produce secondary pyelectasis. Filling defects caused by a tumor projecting into the pelvis are difficult to differentiate against primary epithelial tumors of the renal pelvis, benign papillomas, or herniated intrapelvic daughter cysts (97,

268) . In advanced cases, the pelvis may be completely obliterated occasioning an abrupt termination of contrast medium in the region of the ureteropelvic junction on retrograde pyelograms. The appearance of such lesions simulates nonfunctioning hydronephrosis with obstruction of the ureteropelvic junction. Large

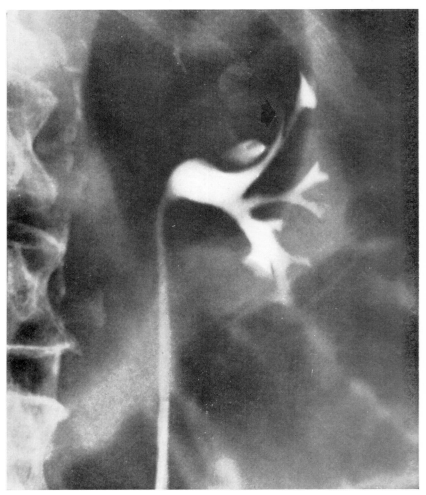

FIGURE 2. A retrograde pyelogram demonstrates displacement of infundibula and calyces of the superior calyceal group of the left kidney by a mass. Amputation of the secondary calyx (arrow) suggests a neoplasm. A tilt of the axis of the kidney reflects predominate medial growth of the tumor.

tumors, particularly if involving the upper or lower pole, may displace the kidney and cause rotation of the kidney axis.

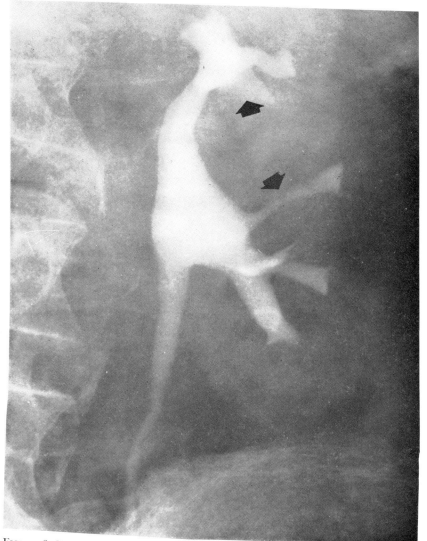

FIGURE 3. Note the displacement and elongation of the infundibulum of the mid calyceal group of the left kidney *(arrow)* and amputation of a secondary calyx of the superior calyceal group indicating the presence of a neoplasm. This infusion pyelogram affords excellent detail demonstration of the pyelocalyceal structures.

Nonfunction of a kidney on intravenous urograms may be seen with renal tumors invading the renal vein. This is usually characterized by a sustained nephrographic stain of the involved kidney (27). Unlike extensive vascular or inflammatory disease, massive tumor usually does not alter renal function. Occasionally a completely normal intravenous urogram may be seen in spite of extensive tumor involvement.

In our experience, a definitive diagnosis of a renal cell carcinoma was established by intravenous and/or retrograde pyelography in only somewhat better than one-third of all patients seen for this lesion (Table VI). Papillary carcinoma of the renal pelvis, conversely, is a lesion that is diagnosable with great accuracy on the intravenous or retrograde urogram (Table VI) (27).

Nephrotomography has greatly enhanced our ability to diagnose neoplasms of the kidney (85). The demonstration of abnormal "tumor-type" vessels within the mass, puddling and irregular opacification of the mass on the arteriographic phase of the nephrotomogram have been advocated as reliable criteria for the diagnosis of a neoplasm (54, 87, 88, 89, 91). The density of the mass greater or equal to that of the adjacent renal parenchyma, irregular opacification of the mass, poorly defined margins of the mass fading into the adjacent normal renal parenchyma are considered dependable criteria for the diagnosis of a solid neoplasm on the nephrographic phase of the nephrotomogram (Table VII) (Fig. 4). The demonstration of a thick or irregular wall around a radiolucent mass on the nephrographic phase nephrotomograms suggests the presence of a cystic or necrotic tumor (16, 37, 218) (Fig. 5). Bosniak et al., emphasized that a wall demonstrated on nephrotomogram thicker than a pencil line is not compatible with a diagnosis of a renal cyst and that, in the presence of any thickened or irregular wall, the diagnosis of a necrotic tumor should be entertained. It should be emphasized that these findings can be simulated by an infected cyst (164, 165).

Considerable controversy exists whether phase nephrotomography is essential for ascertaining a diagnosis (175). The necessity of multiple injections of contrast medium increases the total dosage significantly. The simplified technique of nephrotomography

TABLE VI*

COMPARISON OF DIAGNOSTIC ACCURACY OF VARIOUS ROENTGENOGRAPHIC EXAMINATIONS IN THE
ASSESSMENT OF RENAL MASS LESIONS
(361 CONSECUTIVE PATIENTS)

	Total No.	KUB	IVP and Retrograde Pyelogram	Nephrotomo-gram	Renal Scintiscan	Arteriogram	Cyst Puncture and Aspiration
Benign Cysts	106	2/106	78/106	72/92	17/20	102/106	104/106
Multilocular Cysts	15	0/15	9/15	4/6	4/6	12/12	12/12
Tumor in Cyst	5	0/5	0/5	0/5	0/5	3/5	5/5
Inflammatory Cyst	3	0/3	0/3	1/3	0/3	1/3	3/3
Parapelvic Cyst	8	0/8	2/8	1/5	0/5	6/8	6/6
Hypernephroma	120	0/120	46/120	38/114	7/50	109/120[1]	12/12[1]
Papillary Renal CA	29	0/29	26/29	0/12	0/10	8/14	none performed
Metastatic CA	5	0/5	0/5	0/3	0/3	2/5	1/1
Sarcoma	1	0/1	0/1	0/1	0/1	1/1	none performed
Lymphoma	2	0/2	0/2	0/2	0/1	1/2	none performed
Hamartoma	3	0/3	0/3	0/3	none performed	3/3	none performed
Parapelvic-Lipoma	2	0/2	1/2	2/2	none performed	1/1	none performed
Fibro-Lipoma	1	0/1	0/1	1/1	none performed	1/1	none performed
Adenoma	41	0/41	0/41	1/12	0/10	32/41	0/2
Pyelonephritis	12	1/12	5/12	0/6	0/6	10/12	none performed
Renal TB	2	1/2	2/2	0/2	0/1	1/2	none performed
Polycystic Disease	2	0/2	1/2	2/2	1/2	2/2	none performed
Multicystic Disease	2	0/2	0/2	1/2	0/1	2/2	1/1
Hydronephrosis	2	0/2	2/2	0/1	0/1	1/1	none performed
Accuracy	261	4/361	172/361	123/274	29/123	298/341	144/148
% Accuracy			48%	44½%	24%	87%	97%

[1]Complementing Techniques
*Courtesy, Lang, E.K.—Radiology

CORRECT DIAGNOSIS/TOTAL NUMBER PERFORMED

TABLE VII*

NEPHROTOMOGRAPHIC CRITERIA FOR RENAL CYSTS AND NEOPLASMS

Cyst	Neoplasm
ARTERIAL PHASE Mass avascular	Pathologic vessels, pooling or laking of contrast media in vessels within mass
	Arteriovenous aneurysms
NEPHROGRAPHIC PHASE Mass homogeneously radiolucent throughout	Mass equal or greater density than surrounding parenchyma
Well-defined, thin walls	Necrosis will result in blotchy, irregular poorly defined zones of radiolucency within mass
Sharp demarcation from normal functioning parenchyma	Thick or irregular wall
Acute sharp angle spur formed at junction of cyst wall and cortex	

*Adapted from: Evans, John, M.D.: The accuracy of diagnostic radiology. JAMA 204:131-134, 1968.

utilizing contrast medium administration by drip infusion is now greatly preferred although it permits assessment only in the nephrographic phase (247).

Varying rates of accuracy in the diagnosis of renal cell carcinoma have been claimed for nephrotomography. Chynn and Evans reported an accuracy rate of 94 percent (54) (Table VIII). Witten *et al.* reported an accuracy rate of 89 percent in the diagnosis of renal cell carcinoma by nephrotomography but emphasized the presence of a large number of indeterminate studies raising the margin of error (287). Most authors concur that the accuracy rate is acceptable for those cases demonstrating unequivocal findings of tumor on nephrotomograms. However, a substantial number of indeterminate studies reduces the rate of accurate diagnosis to somewhere in the 70 percent range (37, 218). This observation was confirmed and reiterated by our experience. A definitive correct diagnosis of a hypernephroma was made in only 33 percent of our 114 patients examined by this method with a histologically proven diagnosis of clear cell carcinoma (Table VI). It should be emphasized that all equivocal cases were excluded; this group would otherwise have accounted for another 32 accurate diagnoses. However, on basis of our protocol, a diagnosis was

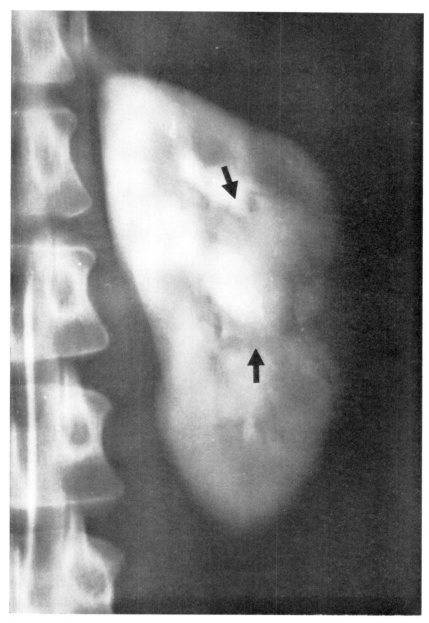

FIGURE 4. The nephrographic phase of the nephrotomogram demonstrates an irregular, mottled opacification of the mass with poorly defined margins fading into the normal renal parenchyma, findings suggesting a solid neoplasm. Areas of necrosis demonstrated on the gross specimen appeared to correlate to the mottled appearance of the mass noted on the nephrotomogram.

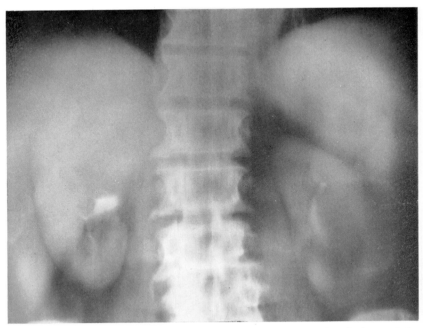

FIGURE 5. The nephrotomogram demonstrates space-occupying lesions of decreased straining quality in the upper pole of the right kidney and in the midportion of the left kidney. Irregular margins of the mass in the upper pole of the right kidney *(arrows)* and a thick wall of the otherwise well demarcated mass in the midportion of the left kidney suggested a cystic hypernephroma. Exploration confirmed the presence of a cystic hypernephroma involving the upper pole of the left kidney; the lesion in the midportion of the right kidney, however, proved to be an infected cyst.

assigned on basis of the respective study only if all criteria for a definitive diagnosis were met (Table VI). The correlation of accuracy of diagnosis based on nephrotomographic criteria versus arteriographic criteria showed that at least in three instances a tumor was diagnosed on basis of a thick-walled avascular lesion which was subsequently proven to be an inflammatory lesion. The nephrotomographic criteria, of ill-defined, irregular wall margins, occasioned the erroneous diagnosis of a tumor in three inflammatory lesions and in one benign cyst (Table IX).

On the basis of these observations, nephrotomography is pri-

TABLE VIII*
ACCURACY OF NEPHROTOMOGRAPHIC DIAGNOSIS*

Diagnosis	No. of Patients	Error Proven by Operation or Autopsy	Percentage of Error
Normal	127	5	4
Renal cysts	203		
Polycystic	37	13	6
	240 cases		
Renal carcinoma	77	5	6
Miscellaneous	56	2	4
including pyelo-nephritis, anomalies, extrarenal mass, renal abscess, etc.			

*From Chynn and Evans, and Southwood and Marshall
**Adapted from Evans, John, M.D.: The accuracy of diagnostic radiology. JAMA 204:131-134, 1968.

TABLE IX*

COMPARATIVE ACCURACY OF CRITERIA ESTABLISHED BY NEPROTOMOGRAPHY VS ARTERIOGRAPHY IN THE DIAGNOSIS OF RENAL MASS LESIONS IN 133 PATIENTS

ARTERIOGRAPHIC CRITERIA \ NEPHROMOGRAPHIC CRITERIA	AVASCULAR	Avascular thin walled	Avascular thick walled	Avascular with ill defined margin	HYPERVASCULAR	Hypervascular
AVASCULAR		49 / 50 \ 1 / 0		0 / 1 \ 1 / 0		
Avascular with abnormal vessels after adrenalin		0 / 5 \ 5 / 0	0 / 2 \ 2 / 0	0 / 1 \ 1 / 0		
Avascular with neovascular pattern in rim		0 / 5 \ 5 / 0	0 / 4 \ 4 / 1	1 / 3 \ 3 / 1		0 / 1 \ 1 / 0
Avascular with collateral vessels		0 / 1 \ 1 / 0	0 / 8 \ 8 / 1	0 / 2 \ 2 / 1		
HYPERVASCULAR						
Hypervascular with homogeneous stain			0 / 1 \ 1 / 1	0 / 3 \ 3 / 1		0 / 6 \ 6 / 1
Hypervascular tumorstain and tumor vessels		0 / 1 \ 1 / 0	0 / 18 \ 18 / 0	0 / 8 \ 8 / 0		0 / 13 \ 13 / 0

Legend for cell quadrants:
TOTAL NO. (left) / CYST (top) \ TUMOR (right) / INFLAMMATORY LESION (bottom)

*Courtesy, Lang, E.K.—Radiology.

marily recommended as a screening technique for the identification of space-occupying lesions and should be used as a definitive diagnostic modality only if all nephrotomographic criteria are met unequivocally and a technically satisfactory nephrotomogram is available for interpretation (232, 247, 263, 284).

The introduction of technetium 99 M pertechnetate and the use of a gamma ray scintillation camera for recording of the early capillary phase has greatly enhanced the diagnostic ability of the renal scintiscanograms for hypernephromas (240). This technique permits identification of increased and abnormal vascularity in a tumor and, therefore, differentiation between neoplasms, cysts or other ischemic lesions. The renal scintiscanogram, performed in the past by injection of radiochlormerodrin was limited in diagnostic capability and could merely demonstrate a space-occupying lesion (30, 127, 151, 202, 260). We have successfully deployed technetium 99 M pertechnetate gamma ray scintiscanograms for the diagnosis of renal tumor in a limited number of patients since the original communication by Rosenthal (240).

The variability of the appearance of the gross specimen of a hypernephroma is reflected on the angiogram (5, 78, 191, 193). The characteristic arteriographic pattern of a hypernephroma consists of a network of irregular vessels of varying caliber (34, 239) (Fig. 6). Aneurysms or arteriovenous shunts are frequently identifiable (1, 138) (Fig. 7). The demonstration of abnormally dilated and tortuous vessels of varying caliber following the perimeter of an expanding lesion is considered diagnostic for hypernephroma. The vascular changes within the tumor are best studied by selective angiography (193). This technique demonstrates the characteristic large, irregular and tortuous vessels within the tumor, many of them ending abruptly. The numerous small arterial and venous branches which may show aneurysmal dilatation and a tendency of sluggish flow or puddling of the injected contrast medium are likewise most easily assessible by this technique. In other areas, rapid shunting of contrast medium through small arteriovenous fistulae may be the characteristic feature often diagnosable only on basis of premature opacification of the veins (1, 138). In some hypernephromas, small capillary vessels predomi-

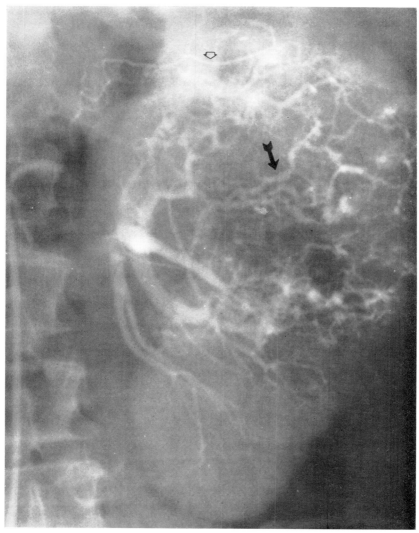

FIGURE 6. A selective renal arteriogram demonstrates the characteristic vascular pattern of a hypernephroma. Note the telltale change in caliber of vessels *(arrow)* and supply derived from the superior capsular artery indicating extension of the tumor into the fat capsule *(small arrow)*.

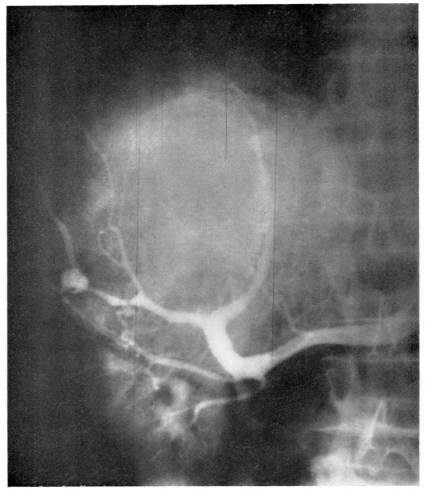

FIGURE 7. The aneurysm at the perimeter of the mass *(arrow)* is one of the typical arteriographic features of a hypernephroma. Note the relative avascularity in the center of the tumor.

nate producing an increased stain visible throughout both arterial and venous phases. This increased stain is best demonstrated on nephrotomograms performed in conjunction with a selective arteriogram (78). However, other hypernephromas may be significantly avascular. Watson, in his series of 100 patients, found 6 tumors to be avascular, 16 to show minimal vascularity, 16 to show moderate vascularity, and 62 to show marked vascularity (276). We found a similar distribution pattern in our series. The avascular tumors do not appear to differ from other tumors as far as demarcation or encapsulation is concerned, however, many appear to have cystic or necrotic centers. Ranniger reported three cases of necrotic hypernephromas in which the angiogram failed to demonstrate tumor vessels entering the renal mass. The correct diagnosis, however, was made on basis of a few small, irregular and tortuous vessels identifiable in the border zone between the mass and the normal parenchyma. These vessels had a decidedly different appearance from the normal but compressed vessels surrounding a renal cyst. A faint but spotty stain was also identifiable on the parenchymal phase of the angiogram. An ill-defined and irregular border between the mass lesion and the functioning renal parenchyma further affirmed the diagnosis (170, 228).

Selective pre-injection of approximately 10μg. of epinephrine hydrochloride in 10 ml of carrier solution into the renal artery has greatly facilitated the demonstration of relatively small tumor vessels in cystic or necrotic tumors (3, 14, 141, 142, 162, 163) (Fig. 8a, b, c). The propensity of normal arteries to contract after exposure to epinephrine results in marked contraction of the entire normal arterial bed of the kidney. Abnormal tumor capillaries fail to respond to epinephrine and, therefore, become more evident (Fig. 17a, b, 20). Kahn *et al.* reported improved visualization of abnormal vessels in renal cell carcinoma in 22 of 24 patients (142). It is, however, emphasized that false negative responses particularly in renal pelvic tumors and metastatic lesions have been reported (142). False positive responses have also been observed in inflammatory lesions and benign renal tumors. Kahn described a positive response of vessels in a benign renal adenoma which thus became indistinguishable from a carcinoma. The vessels of a renal abscess, likewise, showed a positive response to adrenalin hydrochloride and the lesion was erroneously categorized as a tumor (142). We can confirm the latter observation and have noted inconclusive response to epinephrine of small vessels surrounding a renal abscess.

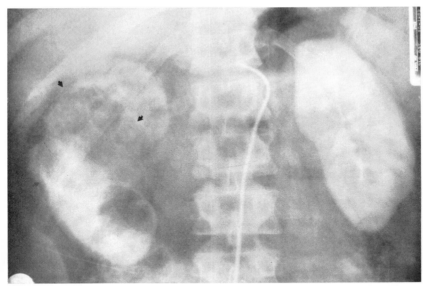

FIGURE 8a, b, c. A flush aortogram demonstrates a relatively avascular lesion in the midportion of the kidney. The selective arteriogram identifies characteristic tumor vessels and an aneurysm within this mass. Injection of 10μg of epinephrine hydrochloride results in constriction of the normal vascular bed and has accentuated opacification of the tumor vessels. This phenomenon has been successfully deployed for selective perfusion or infarction of the tumor with chemotherapeutic agents or radioactive pellets. (Courtesy, Lang — Journal of Urology.)

The demonstrable vascular changes caused by a hypernephroma may be limited to the renal artery bed only or may involve other vessels (78). The flush aortogram has been recommended for assessment of extrarenal vessels. In large tumors, one may observe enlargement of the renal artery supplying the tumor because of increased flow to the tumor and frequently because of the presence of arteriovenous shunts. Large tumors may occasionally displace the main renal artery, the hepatic, pancreatic, and splenic arteries or even the aorta, a finding which is again best demonstrated on flush aortograms.

The necessity of staging of hypernephromas for selection of the optimal choice of therapeutic modality promising control

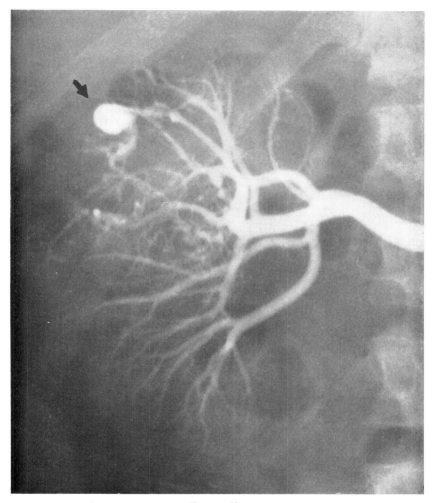

FIGURE 8b.

of the lesion and for an accurate prognostication has increased the
need for a reliable diagnostic technique capable of establishing
the correct stage preoperatively. The arteriogram is superbly capable of filling this demand. A selective renal arteriogram can readily establish the fact that a hypernephroma is confined to the renal
parenchyma. Differentiation of encapsulation versus diffuse infil-

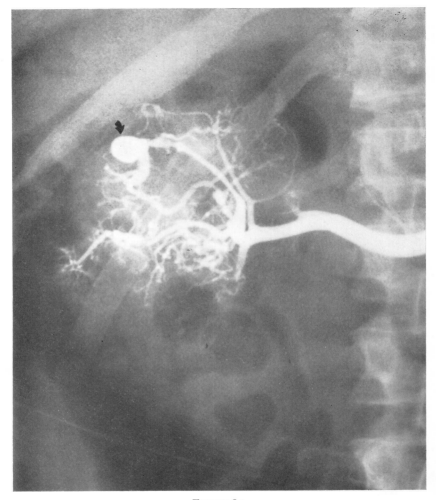

FIGURE 8c.

tration of the margins by tumor can be answered by the arteriogram (Fig. 9) (Table X). The propensity of cortical hypernephromas to derive some of their vascular supply from the capsular
arteries is, likewise, readily demonstrable by selective capsular artery injection (Fig. 10) (112). As long as the vascular supply of a
tumor is derived only from the renal or capsular vessels, it can be

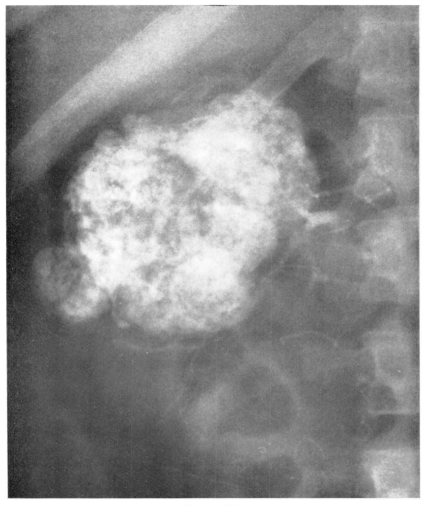

FIGURE 8d.

assumed that the tumor is confined within the renal fat capsule. Documentation of this feature in both AP as well as appropriate oblique projections, however, is mandatory to exclude the possibility of extrarenal vascular supply of the tumor with confidence. If the question of cannibalism of extrarenal vascular supply is

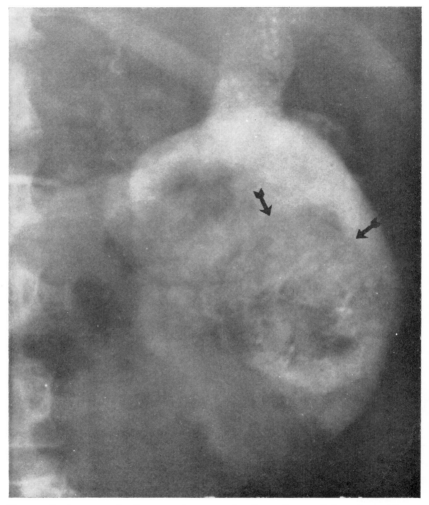

FIGURE 9. A superselective arteriogram of a branch supplying the mid anterior one-third of the left kidney demonstrates a well incapsulated hypernephroma metastasis. Note the sharp demarcation of this lesion against normal renal parenchyma *(arrows)*.

raised on basis of the appearance on the flush injection, or, in patients with ill-defined margins of the tumor, selective renal artery injections and selective arteriographic studies of appropriate

TABLE X*

STAGING OF RENAL CELL CARCINOMA ON BASIS OF ARTERIOGRAPHIC
AND VENOGRAPHIC CRITERIA

I. a. Confined to kidney.	
b. Extension to perirenal fat. (vascular supply limited to renal and capsular arteries)	
II. a. Perirenal extension. (cannibalism of adjacent vascular supply)	
b. Extension into renal vein.	
c. Extension into regional lymph nodes.	
III. a. Extension into inferior vena cava.	
b. Metastases to para-aortic nodes.	
c. Distant metastases. (liver, adrenal, lung, contra-lateral kidney, etc.)	

*Courtesy, Lang, E.K.—Radiology.

neighboring arterial systems are indicated. Selective injection of
the lumbar artery, subcostal artery, phrenic or midadrenal artery
will readily identify cannibalization of their respective vascular

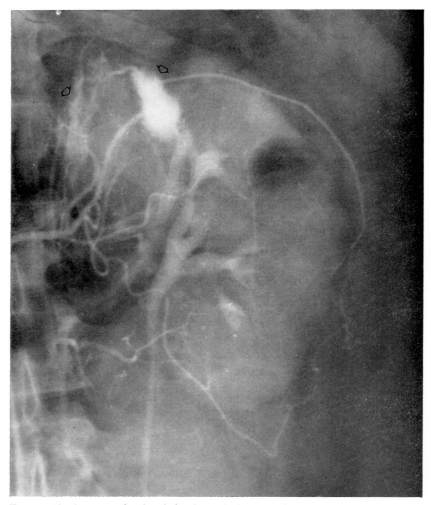

FIGURE 10. A superselective injection of the superior capsular artery of the left kidney demonstrates opacification of the midadrenal branches, the superior and inferior capsular arteries and pelvic branches. Note the abnormal vessels along the medial circumference of the upper pole of the left kidney *(arrows)* and characteristic puddling of dye in this necrotic hypernephroma deriving most of its vascular supply from the capsular arteries.

system by the tumor (Fig. 13, 14a, b, 15). Injection of these vessels with a bolus 4 to 5 cc of contrast medium will demonstrate

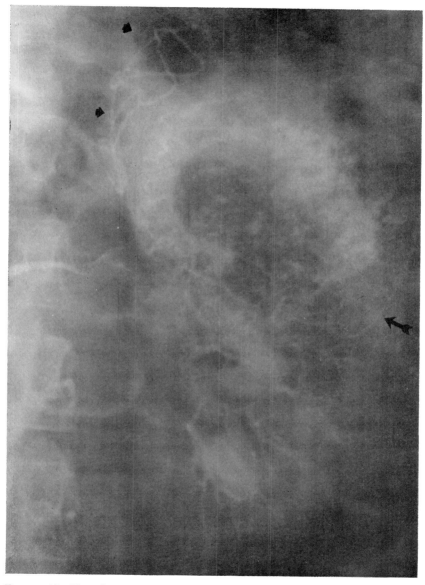

FIGURE 11. Vascular supply from the superior *(arrows)* and midcapsular arteries *(arrows)* indicates extension of this hypernephroma into the renal fat capsule.

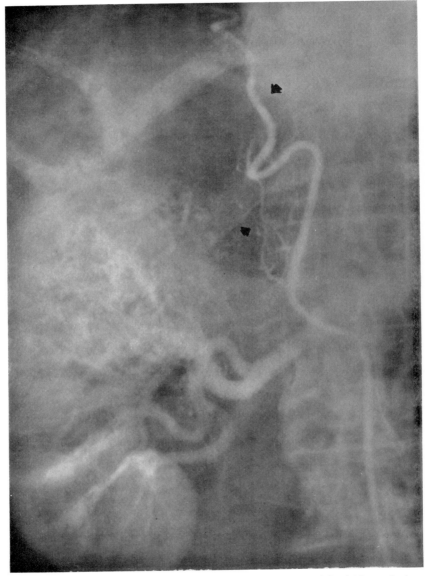

FIGURE 12. A hypernephroma of the upper pole of the right kidney derives some of its supply from the midadrenal artery and from a hugely hypertrophied phrenic artery *(arrows)* indicating direct extension of the tumor into the adrenal and diaphragm.

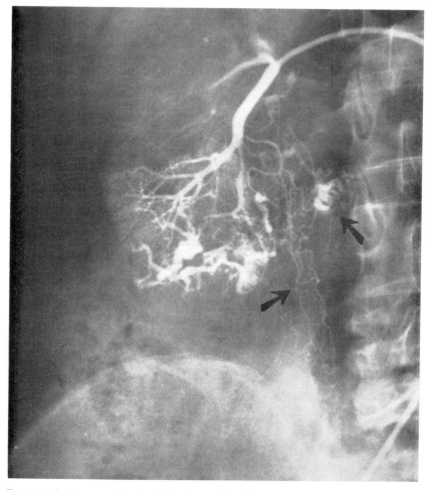

FIGURE 13. A superselective injection of the lower polar branch vessel of the right renal artery demonstrates obvious tumor vessels of a hypernephroma. Note collateral flow to dilated ureteric arteries suggesting the presence of metastatic implants to the ureter as well as to a node *(arrows)*. (Courtesy, Lang — Journal of Urology.)

retrograde flow into the tumor itself and, thus, ascertain tragression of the tumor through the renal capsule. On rare occasions, direct extension of the tumor into structures supplied by the su-

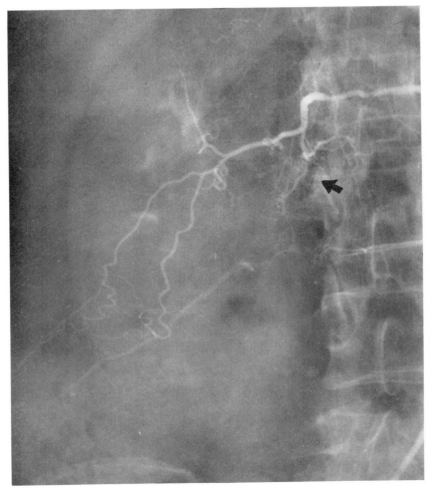

FIGURE 14. A selective injection of the first lumbar artery demonstrates a cluster of abnormal vessels in regional nodes indicating metastatic tumor spread.

perior mesenteric artery or the celiac vessels may be present and appropriate examinations of these vascular systems may then be indicated. Selective hepatic arteriograms, however, should be carried out in all patients in whom metastatic disease is suspected

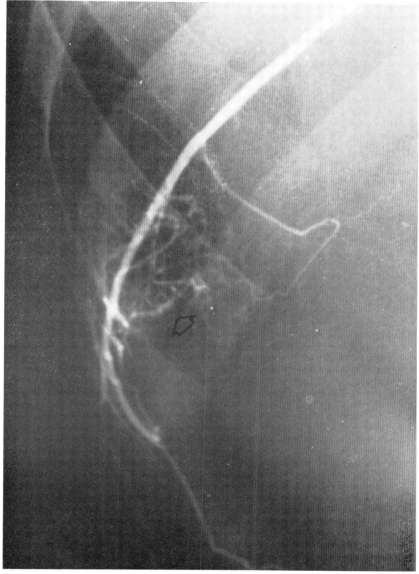

FIGURE 15. A selective injection of a subcostal artery demonstrates a cluster of tumor vessels indicating direct tumor extension to the erector trunci muscle groups. Cannibalism of the arterial system of another organ indicates transgression of the fascial plane by the tumor. (Courtesy, Lang — Radiology.)

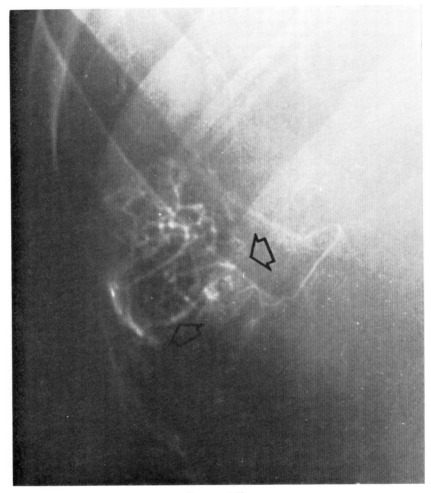

FIGURE 15b.

because of the known predilection of metastatic implants for the liver (141).

Selective renal arteriograms are of paramount importance in the assessment of tumor extension into the renal vein. After the diagnosis of a hypernephroma has been established by arteriography, selective injection of a large bolus of 20 to 30 cc of sodium diatrizoate into the renal artery may be carried out to permit adequate late opacification of the renal vein for assessment of tumor extension or tumor implants (Fig. 16a, b, 17a, b, 18). Retrograde catheterization of the renal vein via the inferior vena cava is not recommended because of the possibility of dislodging tumor fragments and resultant distal embolization. Inferior vena cavography, however, is a safe and useful examination to supplement the information derived from arteriograms and to assess for any possible extension of tumor from the renal vein into the inferior vena cava (Table X, XI) (143).

Extension of a hypernephroma into perirenal structures can also be appraised on retroperitoneal gas studies. If the tumor is contained within the kidney or fat capsule, unimpaired dissectability of the renal margins is demonstrable on the retroperitoneal gas study (Fig. 19). However, if the tumor has invaded adjacent structures, lack of dissectability will be manifest.

We have used arteriographic staging of hypernephromas for the past nine years and found an excellent correlation of arteriographic findings and surgical data and specimen (163, 165). In some instances, the presence of metastatic disease or extension was demonstrated on histopathologic specimen only because of deliberate search based on pre-existing arteriographic knowledge of extension of disease to these structures (6, 38, 39).

In our series of 120 patients, 20 lesions were confined to the renal parenchyma, 7 of these demonstrated encapsulation on arteriograms (Table XI) (Fig. 9). Twenty-two of the lesions derived some of their vascular supply from the capsular artery and, hence, suggested extension of the lesion to the capsule or into the perinephric fat (Fig. 10, 11, 20, 21). Histopathologic examination of these specimen proved tumor in the perivesical fat in 14 of the patients. The remaining 8 demonstrated extension of the tumor to the renal capsule with some arterial supply derived from perforating vessels of the capsular arteries. Twenty-seven of the patients were staged as a IIa lesion because of demonstrable cannibalism of neighboring vascular systems. Tapping into the subcostal artery, lumbar arteries, and phrenic arteries appeared to be the most frequent manifestation of tumor extension into the skele-

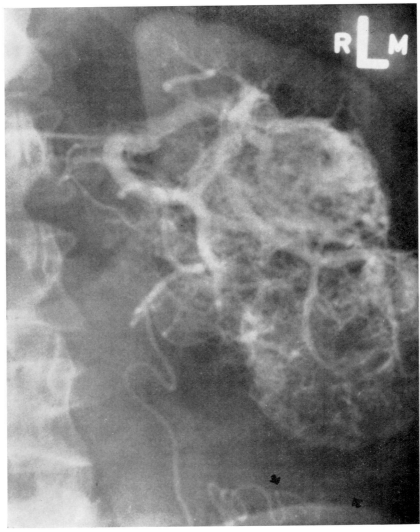

FIGURE 16a, b, c. A selective injection of 30 cc of sodium diatrizoate into the left renal artery demonstrates a huge hypernephroma replacing the entire lower pole and midportion of the left kidney. Note obvious tumor extension into the renal pelvis and renal vein on the late phase roentgenogram. Tortuous collaterals indicate tragression of the tumor along the lower pole into adjacent structures. A roentgenogram of the injected gross specimen demonstrates the hugely dilated renal vein completely replaced by tumor *(arrows)*.

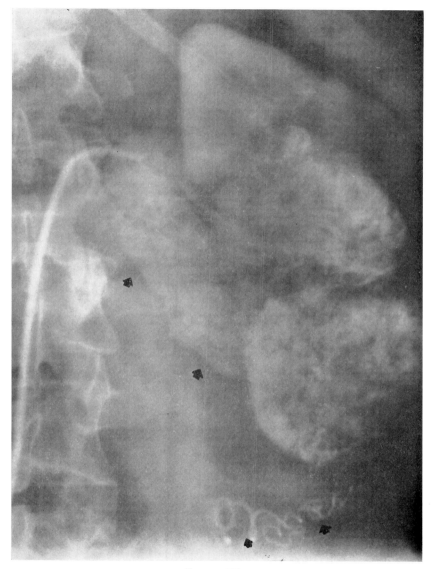

FIGURE 16b.

tal muscles of the retroperitoneal space (Fig. 13, 14a, b, 15, 16). The presence of seeding metastases to the ureters suggested on basis of arteriographic demonstration of enlargement of the ureteral artery was confirmed in 5 of 7 patients in our series (Fig. 13). The two other patients showed tumor extension to the adventitia of the ureter but invasion through its muscularis had not occurred.

Extension of tumor into the renal vein without distant metastases was demonstrated on arteriograms in 12 patients (Fig. 16a, b, c,

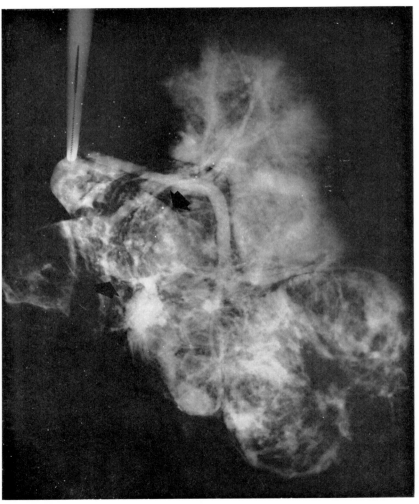

FIGURE 16c.

17a, b). Tumor extension into the renal vein was diagnosed either on basis of a demonstrable tumor mass within the opacified renal vein or its complete occlusion. In 9 of the 12 patients, including all 4 pa-

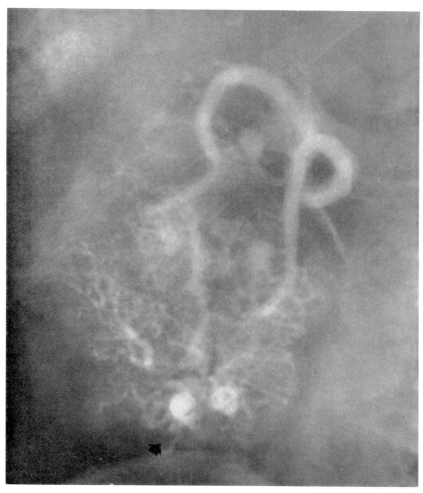

FIGURE 17a, b. A selective renal arteriogram aided by intra-arterial injection of epinephrine demonstrates a huge hypernephroma replacing the lower pole of the right kidney. Aneurysms are demonstrated within the mass *(arrow)*. Thrombosis of the renal vein is suggested on basis of preferential drainage of the tumor to huge retroperitoneal veins *(arrow)* and failure of opacification of the renal vein.

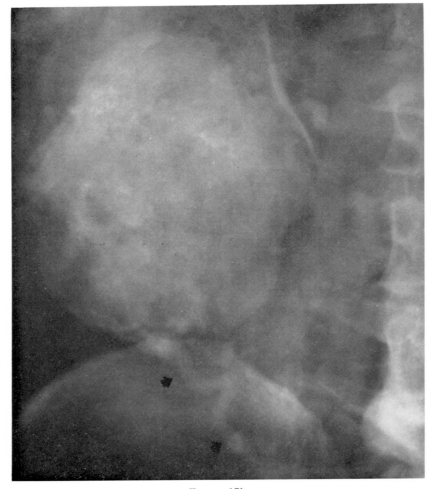

FIGURE 17b.

tients who demonstrated a complete occlusion of the renal vein, abnormal draining veins arising from the periphery of the tumor were demonstrated. However, venous drainage of a tumor via collateral veins to other retroperitoneal structures was observed in 5 patients who exhibited no evidence of renal vein invasion. In these instances, it merely appeared to indicate transgression of the tumor through the renal capsule and tapping of the vascular system of

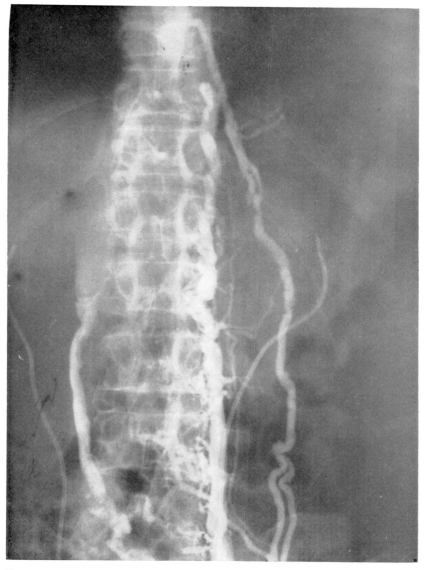

FIGURE 18. An inferior vena cavogram demonstrates collateral flow via the hemiazygous system, the epigastric veins and what appears to be a complete obliteration of the inferior vena cava. These findings indicate massive tumor extension into the inferior vena cava.

TABLE XI*

ARTERIOGRAPHIC FINDINGS AS RELEVANT TO STAGE IN A SERIES
OF 120 PATIENTS WITH RENAL CELL CARCINOMA

STAGE	TOTAL NO		extension of tumor into		
			renal vein	inferior vena cava	paravertebral venous plexus
I. a. (Confined to the kidney).	20				
b. (Extension into fat capsule; vascular supply limited to capsular and renal arteries).	22				
II. a. (Perirenal extension; cannibalism of adjacent vascular supply).	27				
1. Phrenic arteries X		9			
2. Subcostal arteries X		16			
3. Lumbar arteries X		10			
4. Ureteral arteries X		7			
5. Adrenal arteries X		2			
6. Pancreatico-duodenal arteries X		1			
7. Splenic arteries X		1			
b. (Extension into renal vein).	12				
c. (Extension to regional lymph nodes).	13				
III. a. (Extension into inferior vena cava)	3				
1 (associated with renal vein extension)		3			
b. (Metastases to para-aortic nodes)	3				
1 (associated with regional node involvement)		3			
c. (Distant metastases)	20				
1. Liver X		12	12	10	5
2. Adrenal X		11	6	3	1
3. Lung X		3	3	2	0
4. Contra-lateral kidney X		7	5	3	2
5. CNS X		2	2	2	2
6. Osseous structures X		5	4	3	3

X   OFTEN   MULTIPLE   INVOLVEMENT

*Courtesy, Lang, E.K.—Radiology.

perirenal structures (184). The normal appearance of the renal vein eliminates the possibility of renal vein thrombosis or invasion by tumor (80.) Failure of visualization of the renal vein following injection of small amounts of contrast medium, 8 to 10 cc, however does not permit the conclusion that one may be dealing with tumor occlusion of the renal vein (80, 276). Watson emphasized that only a small percentage of his patients in whom the renal vein failed to opacify adequately demonstrated evidence of gross or

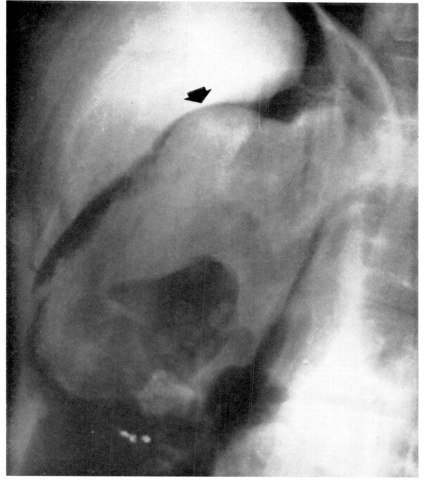

FIGURE 19. A retroperitoneal gas study demonstrates a protuberance along the upper pole of the right kidney. Unimpaired dissectability of the renal margin suggests that this neoplasm is contained within the renal capsule.

microscopic tumor invasion of the renal vein. He confirmed our impression that the demonstration of collateral veins draining a tumor does not necessarily suggest obstruction of the renal vein (80, 276).

A stage IIc lesion was suggested in 13 patients on basis of a suspicious tumor blush in the region of regional lymph nodes (Table XI). At least 4 of the patients demonstrated abnormal corkscrew vessels and puddling of contrast medium similar to the pattern seen in the primary tumor. Lymphangiography performed via lymphatics of the dorsum of the forefoot does not usually visualize regional lymph nodes of the kidney. Not infrequently, even metastases to para-aortic nodes may be missed. In our own experience, lymphangiography has not significantly contributed to stag-

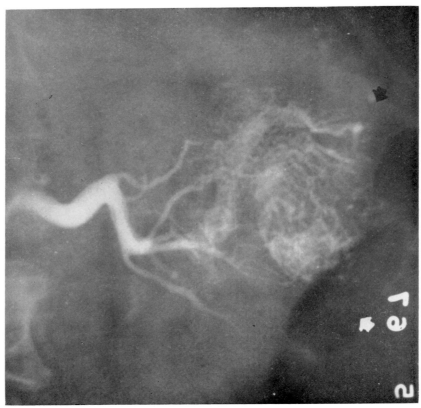

FIGURE 20. A selective renal arteriogram precluded by injection of 10μg of adrenalin hydrochloride demonstrates abnormal vessels in the midportion of the right kidney extending through the capsule. Note the cannibalism of the midcapsular artery by this tumor indicating extension into the perirenal fat *(white arrows)*. (Courtesy, Lang — Radiology.)

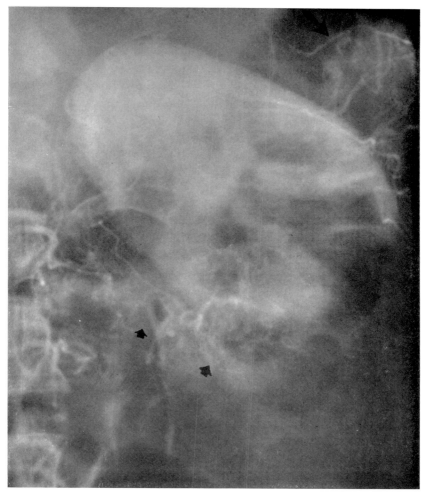

FIGURE 21. Simultaneous selective injections of the superior capsular artery and the second lumbar artery demonstrate opacification of tumor extending into the hilum of the kidney with supply predominately from the lumbar and midcapsular artery *(arrows)* and of tumor extension along the lateral circumference of the kidney with supply from the superior capsular artery *(arrow)*. The known propensity of the second lumbar artery to give rise to branches communicating with the pelvic and midcapsular arteries precludes against a diagnosis of tumor extension into the retroperitoneal muscles. (Courtesy, Lang — Radiology.)

ing and assessment of metastatic hypernephroma implants and we, therefore, rely on the demonstration of an arteriographic stain or abnormal vessels in these lymph nodes. (Fig. 13).

Extension of tumor to the inferior vena cava without other metastic disease was found in three patients. All three of these patients showed tumor involvement of the renal vein (Fig. 18).

In three of our patients, metastases to para-aortic nodes were diagnosed (Table XI). An arteriographic stain identified metastatic tumor in each patient, however, in two of the patients the diagnosis was further aided by demonstration of a nodular para-aortic mass on retroperitoneal gas studies.

Distant metastases were identified in 20 patients of our series. Metastases to the liver, adrenal and to the contralateral kidney appeared to be most common. It was of interest to note that all patients with metastases to the liver showed renal vein involvement and the majority showed extension of the tumor into the inferior vena cava. The percentage of renal vein involvement was also high with metastases to the adrenal and the contralateral kidney.

The difficulty of differentiating direct tumor extension into the adrenal from a metastatic implant to the adrenal can be abated by use of the arteriogram. Contiguous vascular supply of a tumor mass, involving both kidney and adrenal, by both renal arteries and adrenal vessels serves as proof that direct extension of the tumor into the adrenal or vice versa has occurred (Fig. 22a, b, c). If, however, the tumor in the adrenal derives its vascular supply exclusively from the appropriate vessels of the adrenal, this can be interpreted as conclusive evidence for a metastatic tumor implant (Fig. 23). As in our experience, this will frequently be accompanied by demonstrable tumor invasion of the renal vein or inferior vena cava.

Demonstration of abnormal venous drainage into the paravertebral venous plexus was demonstrated in 13 patients with distant metastases. With the notable exception of metastases to the adrenal, the combination of demonstrable tumor extension to the renal vein or demonstrable abnormal venous drainage to the paravertebral plexus would adequately explain the route for seeding of metastases.

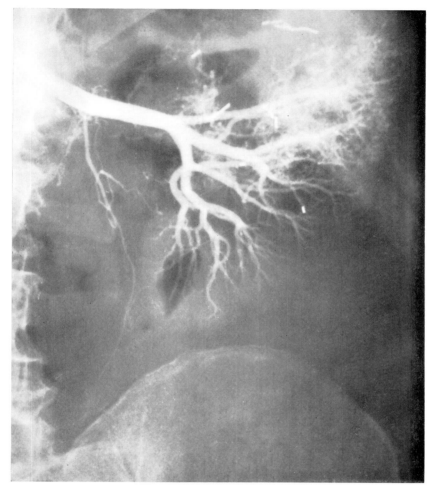

FIGURE 22a, b, c. A selective injection of the main renal artery demonstrates abnormal tumor vessels in the upper one-half of the left kidney and a marked tilt of the kidney axis. A selective injection of a hugely dilated midadrenal artery readily demonstrates tumor which appears to extend directly from the upper pole of the kidney into the adrenal. Note supply of this tumor by a hugely dilated superior capsular artery *(white arrow)* and the phrenic artery *(black arrow)*. Metallic densities within the tumors represent a radioactive infarct implant. Contiguous supply of the tumor by both the midadrenal and renal arteries suggests direct extension of the tumor into the adrenal rather than a metastatic implant. (Courtesy, Lang — Journal of Urology.)

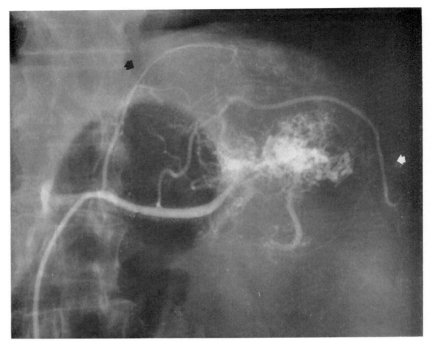

FIGURE 22b.

The significance of arteriographic staging for prognostication and choice of therapeutic modality is well established. Patients with an arteriographic stage I lesion showed a 60 percent 5-year survival in our series. Patients with an arteriographic stage IIa lesion showed a 50 percent 5-year survival, IIb lesions a 25 percent 5-year survival, and IIc lesions an 11 percent 5-year survival. Lesions staged as IIIa, b, c, or d averaged only a 10 percent 5-year survival (Table III).

The value of arteriographic information on hypernephromas when considering a partial nephrectomy has been pointed out by Frimann-Dahl (103). He used partial nephrectomy as treatment for five malignant tumors and angiography was essential for this decision. This principle is directly transferable to the treatment of renal cell carcinoma in a solitary or sole-functioning kidney or

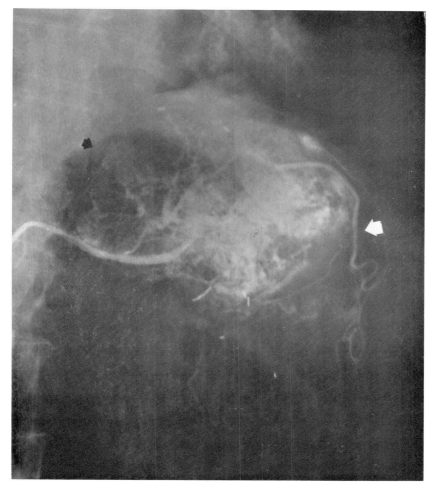

FIGURE 22c.

to the management of simultaneous bilateral carcinoma (3, 255, 258).

Renal arteriography is also pertinent to follow-up examination of surgically removed hypernephromas, for assessment of new metastases or documentation of regression of metastases under radiation or chemotherapeutic management (242).

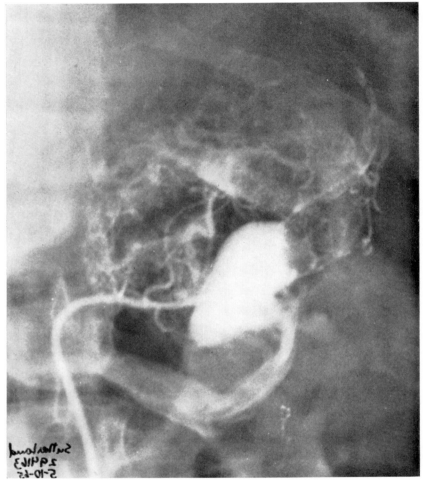

FIGURE 23. A selective injection of the left midadrenal artery demonstrates abnormal vessels in the left adrenal characteristic of the pattern seen with hypernephroma. A clear demarcation of this tumor against the upper pole of the left kidney indicates a metastatic implant to the adrenal from a primary hypernephroma of the opposite kidney.

The accuracy of arteriographic diagnosis and staging of hypernephromas depends on the quality of the technique, selectivity of injection, and completeness of roentgenographic recording. Arteriography is credited with an accuracy of about 95 percent in the diagnosis of hypernephromas and in the differentiation of renal mass lesions (78, 144, 162, 163, 165, 193, 228, 285). In our own series, the arteriogram established a definitive and accurate diagnosis in approximately 90 percent of the patients. However, in combination with cyst puncture, aspiration and double contrast cyst studies deployed in questionable cases, the accuracy rose to 99 percent (Table VI).

Avascular or hypovascular lesions are difficult to assess by arteriography (26). Transitional cell carcinoma, necrotic clear cell carcinoma, and metastatic carcinoma to the kidney are lesions which may simulate benign cysts on arteriograms (26). Cyst puncture, aspiration and double contrast study of cysts, however, will disclose the true nature of these lesions with definity.

Inflammatory cysts, xanthogranulomatous pyelonephritis, renal abscesses, fibrolipomatosis, and hypertrophied parenchyma or local nodular areas of residual normal parenchyma in a chronic pyelonephritic kidney have been confused with hypernephromas on renal arteriograms. Cyst puncture, aspiration and double contrast studies will readily diagnose inflammatory cysts. The characteristic findings of xanthogranulomatous pyelonephritis and fibrolipomatosis will be discussed in detail in a later chapter; suffice it to say that characteristic findings on arteriogram permit differentiation against hypernephroma. Hypertrophied parenchyma or areas of residual normal parenchyma in pyelonephritic kidneys show normal arcuate arteries within the nodules and demonstrable deviation of neighboring interlobar arteries around the hypertrophied segments (149). An intense parenchymal blush on the capillary phase roentgenogram identifies the residual normal or hypertrophied parenchyma in chronic atrophic pyelonephritis. Abnormal tumor vessels, puddling of contrast material and, particularly, early venous filling are conspicuously absent and help confirm the diagnosis.

Pseudotumors of the kidney caused by intraparenchymal hemorrhage often occasioned by prolonged anticoagulation therapy may likewise simulate a necrotic hypernephroma. Although a thick walled and irregular staining capsule can be mimicked by the compressed parenchyma both on nephrotomograms and arteriograms, absence of abnormal vessels and a normal venous phase permit differentiation and a definitive diagnosis (259). The consensus of the recent literature affirms the indispensable position of renal arteriography in the assessment of renal cell carcinoma (193). Its use extends not only to primary diagnosis of the lesion but also to staging and assessment of the extent of the tumor and has recently been advocated as a substitute for biopsy and histopathologic examination in the evaluation of metastatic lesions (38).

BENIGN RENAL TUMORS

Benign parenchymal tumors are relatively rare and therefore of only minor clinical importance. Most of them are small and they rarely reach sufficient size (2 cm in diameter or greater) to be recognized clinically (58). Of those which reach a size large enough to produce clinical signs and symptoms, the overwhelming majority are adenomas, lipomas, or myomas (7, 10, 120, 131, 155, 169).

Histologically, adenomas of the renal cortex are of three types: papillary, alveolar, and tubular (264). The majority of renal adenomas are asymptomatic and are discovered accidentally during clinical investigation for other purposes. Only on rare occasions will these tumors present with symptoms of pain and hematuria. The urographic features are alteration of the renal contour and, as the tumor enlarges, stretching, displacement and elongation of the calyces (192, 194, 199). Absence of destruction of secondary calyces permits differentiation against hypernephroma. Nephrotomography demonstrates a radiolucent mass lesion with a thick and irregular wall, a finding allegedly characteristic for renal adenomas (227). Rabinowitz *et al.* postulated that the opacification of the wall was related to stasis within the capsular venous channels. In our experience, the nephrotomographic appearance is indistinguishable from that of a necrotic hypernephroma. The arteriogram demonstrates stretching and displacement of relatively small arteries around a mass into which only a few perpendicular branches enter. Absence of corkscrew vessels, arteriovenous fistulae and abnormal vessels manifesting changes of caliber permits differentiation from a hypernephroma. However, differentiation against a small solid hypernephroma is difficult on basis of both arteriography and nephrotomography. Even the response of vessels to epinephrine is not reliable in differentiation of these lesions. Kahn reported one case with a false positive epinephrine response in a histologically proven adenoma (142).

Mesenchymal tumors such as fibroma present as a relatively avascular space-occupying lesion with noninvasive characteristics on arteriogram, but generally defy diagnosis by roentgenographic studies (253). Lipomas may be diagnosable on roentgenograms on basis of their relative radiolucency. Parapelvic lipomas, in particular, are easily demonstrable on nephrotomograms (174). The telltale vascular pattern of renal angiomas permits ready arteriographic diagnosis (7, 74). Duckett reported successful preoperative diagnosis of two patients with renal angiomas by selective renal angiograms and described their characteristic vascular pattern.

Angiolipomas are a relatively common lesion and two distinct types are encountered (4, 93, 109, 150, 207, 225, 289). The common hamartoma of mixed mesenchymal origin is multiple and found in patients with tuberous sclerosis. A different, and rare, characteristically unifocal and quiet large angiomyolipoma, not associated with tuberous sclerosis, is found in females in their third to fifth decade of life (183). Hematuria and pain occasioned by the presence of a large mass may occasionally herald the presence of such a tumor (250). Such large tumors may rupture and massive retroperitoneal hemorrhage may result (179, 214, 271). Although it has been suggested by some authors that angiomyolipomas may be diagnosed on the plain roentgenogram by virtue of their striking radiolucency, the validity of this observation is seriously questioned by most authorities (4, 147, 250). There is general agreement in the literature that the urographic findings merely indicate the presence of a mass. Radiolucent areas are not well demarcated and require careful search to be seen at all. The difficulty in identifying the characteristic radiolucency of fat is attributed to the peculiar distribution of fat in these large tumors (4, 283).

Arteriographic demonstration of microaneurysms without evidence of arteriovenous fistulae has been proposed as the diagnostic criterion for angiomyolipomas (27). However, the ability to assuredly identify such a minute characteristic has been questioned by most authors. The striking similarity of the vascular pattern of angiomyolipoma and of renal cell carcinoma has been cited in the literature (183, 195, 276).

The similarity of the arteriographic pattern seen with solid clear cell carcinoma, hamartoma, and renal abscess has been emphasized (27, 185, 188). Cysts, tubular or papillary adenomas, fibromas, lipomas and mesenchymomas, adult unilateral polycystic disease, healing abscesses, pyelonephrosis, tuberculosis in a late healing stage, fibrolipomatosis, xanthogranulomatous pyelonephritis, tumor occurring in cysts, avascular clear cell carcinoma, and transitional cell carcinoma with parenchymal invasion demonstrate the pattern of an avascular mass lesion similar in appearance both on arteriograms and nephrotomograms (27, 71, 195).

Xanthogranulomatous pyelonephritis should be considered in differential diagnosis of any nonfunctioning kidney with hydronephrosis, associated urolithiasis, and deformity of the pyelocalyceal system of the contralateral kidney compatible with pyelonephritis (113, 174, 187). The xanthogranulomatous pyelonephritic kidney may be either smaller than normal or may be intrinsically enlarged and is frequently associated with a perinephric abscess (111, 273). However the lipid laden macrophages fail to yield diagnostic radiolucencies on plain films or angiograms (44). Selective renal arteriograms demonstrate stretching of the segmental arteries and attenuation and lack of normal peripheral arborization. The lack of a definable arterial and nephrographic phase transition is considered characteristic for this entity. Scant and irregular stains, poorly demarcated, are noticed throughout the mass reflecting the presence of residual renal parenchyma with normal staining capacity. Benign neovascularity supplied from extrarenal sources, particularly ureteral arteries and pelvic arteries, reflects response to infection, ischemia, and diminution of the overall blood flow to the kidney. The differentiation against an avascular hypernephroma is possible on basis of absence of abnormal tumor vessels, arterio-venous shunts, aneurysms, and the characteristic puddling of contrast medium.

CHAPTER III

RENAL CYSTIC DISEASE

A LTHOUGH RENAL CYSTS were once considered a very rare and uncommon lesion, recent autopsy series have proven that renal cysts are by far the most common space-occupying lesion involving the kidneys (41). Renal cysts have been found in 3 to 5 percent of all routine autopsies and an incidence rate of diagnosable benign cysts of 2 percent has been claimed for routine intravenous urograms (33). The well established fact that cysts are most common in adults in the fifth and sixth decades has given support to the theory that cysts are acquired rather than congenital (102, 103).

A classification of renal cystic disease based on the etiology and nature of the principal disturbance leading to the formation of cysts has been successfully correlated by Grossman to the functional alterations manifested on the excretory urogram (118) (Table 10 and 12). The classification is broad enough in scope to permit incorporation of various other theories advanced for the explanation of the formation of cysts. Reflecting the complexity of renal organogenesis, Grossman distinguished four types of cystic disease. The first type is characterized by hyperplasia and generalized dilatation of the collecting tubules with a normal nephron. Infantile sponge kidney, medullary sponge kidney, and renal tubular ectasia are the classical clinical representatives of this group. The second type shows a cystic dilatation of the terminal portions of collecting tubules and a complete or nearly complete nephron agenesis. Multicystic kidney, renal dysplasia, multilocular cysts, and simple cysts are the clinical corellaries. The third type is distinguished by cyst formation in the nephrons as well as the collecting tubules. Functioning and functionless nephrons are intermixed. Polycystic disease of the kidney and hamartomas associated

TABLE XII*
CLASSIFICATION OF CYSTIC DISEASE OF THE KIDNEY

Pathologic Entity	IVP Manifestations
Type I	
Infantile sponge kidney (Hamartomatous kidney, polycystic kidneys of the newborn, microcystic kidney disease) Medullary sponge kidney Renal tubular ectasia with congenital hepatic fibrosis	Contrast material in dilated collecting tubules
Type II	
Multicystic kidney Hypoplastic (dysgenetic) cystic kidney Multilocular cysts Simple cysts Hereditary medullary cystic disease (juvenile nephronophthisis)	Nonfunction throughout or in part of kidney; contour changes in renal outline and collecting system
Type III	
Adult polycystic kidneys Tuberous sclerosis	Deformity of renal pelvis and calyces by cysts intermixed with normally functioning tissue
Type IV	
Posterior urethral valves Other obstructions in urethra Urethral obstruction	Small cortical and/or medullary cysts secondary to distal urinary tract obstruction

*Adapted from Grossman, Herman, M.D., *et al.*: Roentgenographic classification of renal cystic disease. Radiology 104:319-331, 1968.

with tuberous sclerosis are the clinical entities assigned to this group. The fourth type is characterized by microscopic subcapsular cyst formation secondary to distal urinary tract obstruction. This entity has been found associated with posterior urethral valves or other urethral obstruction.

While this classification will satisfy demands for a pathological categorization, it is obvious that etiologies other than investigal nephron agenesis with resulting dilatation of the terminal portions of the collecting tubules could result in cyst formation (19, 36, 43). Hepler's experiments proved that cysts could be produced by ligating tubules while, at the same time, occluding the vascular supply (130). Cicatricial changes secondary to vascular or inflammatory disease or obstruction by distal tumor are capable of producing cysts. Andersen attributed narrowing of the neck of some of the cysts to inflammatory fibrosis and, therefore, termed the condition "localizing obliterating pyelonephritis" (8) . These pyelonephritic cysts are quite rare and are, in general, too small to interfere with the renal vascular pattern (124) . Williams reviewed the entire admission material to the department of urology at the London Hospital from 1960 to 1967 and established an incidence rate for pyelonephritic cysts of 0.15 percent (282) . Watkins described a similar type of pyelonephritic cyst which appeared to grow larger in spite of a patent communication to the renal pelvis. He advanced the theory that these rare types of cysts arise as a hydrocalycosis and suggested that some solitary cysts might have originally had a communication with the pelvis which closed at a later date (275) . The similarity of the appearance of a pyelonephric cyst communicating to the renal pelvis or calyces and a cortical cyst communicating to the calyces or pelvis following traumatic rupture is emphasized. Differentiation of these entities on basis of their roentgenographic or even pathologic anatomical appearance might meet with great difficulty (22, 35, 40, 230) .

The etiology of parapelvic cysts has been attributed to obstruction of lymphatic vessels and will be discussed in detail in a later chapter (73) .

SIMPLE RENAL CYSTS

Simple renal cysts are by far the most common form of cyst found in the kidney. They are usually solitary and unilateral. Multiple cysts of this type, however, may occur in one or both kidneys. Occasionally, simple cysts may be situated almost entirely extrarenally; they are then referred to as capsular cysts. The size of simple renal cysts varies widely (50, 64, 104, 112, 173, 180, 220, 267, 275, 277, 288) .

The lower pole of the kidney appears to be the preferential site for renal cysts (102, 103, 154) . Frimann-Dahl found 50 percent of the cysts in the lower pole, 30 percent in the midportion and 20 percent in the upper pole; a similar distribution pattern is reflected in most articles attempting tabulation by location of cysts. An analysis of our composite pathologic and radiologic experience revealed 210 cysts located in the lower pole, 72 in the upper pole, 19 in the mid portion, and 41 multiple lesions in a total series of 342 cysts. Much controversy exists as to whether or not the left kidney is a site of predilection for cysts. Wise found 41 cysts on the left and 30 on the right side (285). Lalli, however, found 17 on the right and only 15 on the left. In our own series, 189 cysts were encountered on the left, 153 on the right. A significant statistical difference in location of renal cysts in the right or left kidney does not appear to exist.

The clinical diagnosis of renal cysts is extremely difficult (57). Hoffman suggested that a palpable mass was more frequently found with cysts than tumors (133). Whether or not a cyst presents as a palpable mass, obviously depends on its size. Pain and hypertension have been associated in about the same frequency with renal cysts as tumors. Hematuria, while admittedly more frequent with renal tumors, may be seen with renal cysts. Gregg found hematuria in 50 percent of his patients with carcinoma and in 33 percent of the patients with renal cysts (115). However, in general urologic practice, hematuria, per se, would by far more frequently indicate the presence of prostatitis, cystitis, or inflammatory disease. Normal urinary beta glucuronidase levels, normal erythrocite sedimentation rate, and absence of anemia would support the diagnosis of cyst over tumor in patients with a known renal mass (114, 133, 246). The findings on the plain roentgenogram depend on the location and the size of the cyst. If the cyst is situated mainly outside the kidney, a well defined round or oval-shaped mass projects from the main mass of the kidney or appears to be directly adjacent to the kidney (Fig. 33a, b). If the cyst, however, is partially imbedded in renal parenchyma, a bulge in the outline of the kidney, reflecting the size of the cyst, may be appreciated. The closer the cyst is located to the surface, the more prominent the bulge. Small intrarenal cysts may produce no demonstrable roentgenographic changes. It has been repeatedly emphasized in the literature that cysts of the lower pole of the kidney cause a characteristic blurring of the psoas shadow. On basis of our experience, this observation can not be confirmed; only unusually large cysts arising from the medial circumference of the lower pole of the kidney may occasionally cause blurring of the psoas shadow. Multiple cysts in close proximity to each other may occasion a coarse lobulation of the contour of the kidney. The claim that cysts may be detected on plain roentgenograms as an area of decreased density has to be rejected emphatically. Since parenchyma and cyst fluid are isodense to the commonly used radiation spectrum, an image of differentiable density is not cast. Only in extremely rare instances, high fat content of the cyst fluid may, indeed, cause a radiolucent appearance. The identification of calcifications in a renal mass, however, deserves special attention and can be a determinate aid in establishing the diagnosis.

CALCIFICATIONS IN RENAL MASS LESIONS

Calcifications in a renal mass may represent dystrophic calcifications in tumor, calcifications in an area of inflammation and necrosis, calcifications in cyst walls, and suspended calcium in calyceal diverticula or cysts. Scattered and mottled dystrophic calcifications are more frequently seen in renal tumors. However, many observers have cautioned against rendering a diagnosis of a renal cyst on basis of a crescent-shaped calcification (47, 52, 72, 243, 262) (Fig. 24, 25). Shockman reported ring-shaped renal calcifications in two tumors and two renal cysts, in an equal occurrence rate (252). Crescent-, ring- or shell-like calcifications may also occur in hydatid disease (66). Deliveliotis *et al.* demonstrated such calcifications in 7 of 12 patients with proven hydatid disease. The final differentiation of a hydatid cyst versus a simple cyst relies on the Casoni test (66).

Ring-shaped calcifications have also been described in Bilharziasas (13). The calcifications in this disease are formed in heavy infiltrates in the renal capsule and, therefore, conform to the renal capsule.

Calcifications in renal cysts, are percentage-wise less frequent than calcifications in renal tumors (72, 222). Phillips reviewed the incidence of calcifications in 225 renal mass lesions. In simple cysts, calcifications occurred in 3 percent of the patients, in polycystic disease in 6 percent, in renal carcinoma in 14 percent, and in neuroblastoma in 53 percent of the patients (222) (Table 4).

The presence of calcifications in tumors has been regarded by most observers as an ominous prognostic sign. Schreiber found

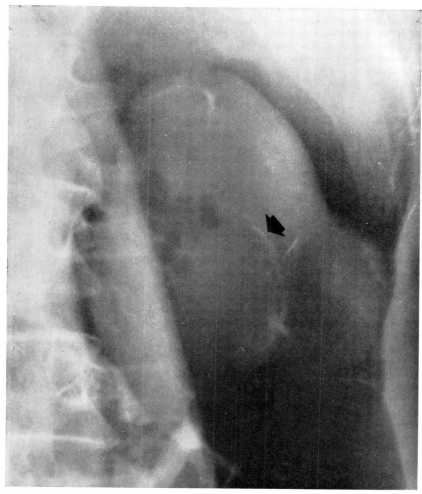

Figure 24. Multiple crescentic calcific shadows indicate the presence of multiple cysts. The concomitant use of a retroperitoneal gas study provides optimal roentgen-physical conditions for demonstration of faint calcific shadows.

calcifications in 22 percent of his patients with renal cell carcinoma. The presence of calcifications was associated with an increase in the likelihood of unresectability from 21 to 29 percent (248). This observation was confirmed by our series. Although calcifications were demonstrated in only 2 of our 120 patients with hypernephromas on the preoperative roentgenograms, specimen roentgenograms utilizing a low kilovoltage, high MAS technique and industrial type "M" film revealed fine punctate calcifications

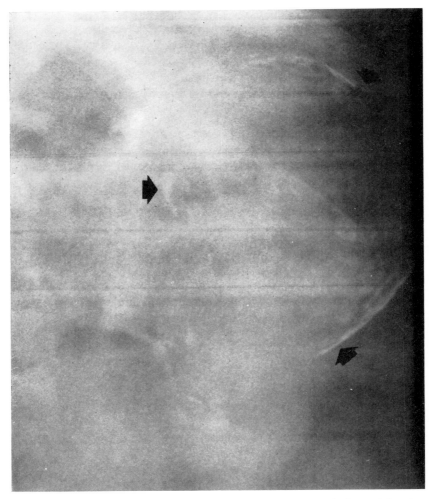

FIGURE 25. Coarse crescentic shadows delineate a huge mass lesion originating from upper one-half of the left kidney. The coarse nature of the calcification favors a neoplasm. This is further supported by the presence of dystrophic and mottled calcifications within the tumor. This case examplifies the fallacy of establishing the diagnosis of a cyst on basis of crescentic calcifications.

in another 27 of 108 specimen thus examined. The percentile 5-year survival of the patients with such fine punctate calcifications on the specimen roentgenograms was significantly decreased compared to those patients lacking demonstrable calcifications on the specimen roentgenograms.

The roentgenographic demonstration of a "suspension" of calcium particles layering in a cystic cavity readily establishes the diagnosis of "milk of calcium" in a cyst or calyceal diverticulum (29, 128, 201). The horizontal layering of "milk of calcium" in a cystic structure demonstrable in upright and decubitus positions differentiates this entity against all other calcifications. Apparent decrease of "milk of calcium" in such cysts has been noted on serial follow-up films suggesting a communication to the pyelocalyceal system (135). Increasing opacification of the cyst during an intravenous pyelogram again alludes to a possible communication with the collecting system (29, 201).

PYELOGRAPHIC CHANGES OCCASIONED BY RENAL CYSTS

The pyelographic changes occasioned by renal cysts depend on the site and size of the lesions. Cortical cysts growing away from the kidney may not deform the renal pelvis and calyces. However, cysts situated deep within the renal parenchyma cause distortion and deformity of calyces, infundibula and the renal pelvis. Lack of distortion of minor calyces by a lesion causing deformity of the infundibula, major calyces, and renal pelvis has been considered pathognomonic for a renal cyst (57). This criterion has been advocated for differentiation of cysts against other space-occupying lesions such as tumors and abscesses (83). Recent reports and our own experience, however, emphasize that while renal cysts usually occasion crescentic deformity, displacement, elongation, and flattening of the major calyces, complete obliteration of major or minor calyces, and irregular distortion and even destruction of minor calyces may occur sometimes with simple cysts (76, 163) (Fig. 26). Differentiation of cysts and renal tumors or inflammatory lesions of the kidney on basis of pyelographic changes cannot be made with a high degree of confidence. Depending on the site and size of the lesion, renal cysts may mimic the changes hith-

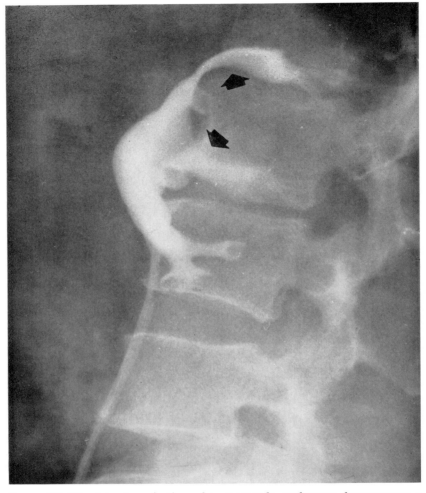

FIGURE 26. The lateral projection of a retrograde pyelogram demonstrates a typical crescentic deformity and splaying of the infundibula of the mid- and superior calyceal group. There is no evidence of destruction of the minor calyces. This type of deformity is considered typical for renal cyst.

erto held pathognomonic for renal tumors. Flattening or crescentic deformity of the medial border of the pelvis is often seen with large renal cysts (97). Large renal cysts may also occasion rotation of the kidney along its perpendicular or transverse axis.

The nephrographic phase of the intravenous pyelogram demonstrates a decreased stain of the renal cyst compared to the surrounding normal renal parenchyma. Larger amounts of contrast medium or infusion pyelograms may be employed to accentuate this difference in staining quality.

Intravenous urography, infusion intravenous urography, and retrograde pyelography are primarily employed for the identification of space-occupying lesions in the kidney without attempting to differentiate the type of renal mass lesion.

NEPHROTOMOGRAPHY IN ASSESSMENT OF RENAL CYSTS

Evans *et al.* first popularized nephrotomography as a diagnostic modality for the assessment of renal masses in 1954 (87). Nephrotomography is basically a form of intravenous renal angiography combined with body section roentgenography (tomography). After an initial enthusiastic acceptance of this technique, mounting reports of errors in differentiation of renal cysts and tumors caused many radiologists to abandon this examination. Statistical reassessment of the diagnostic capability of nephrotomography after addition of new diagnostic criteria established its sphere in the diagnostic armamentarium for assessment of renal mass lesions (37, 54, 88, 89, 90, 91, 163, 257, 287).

The original criteria for the diagnosis of a renal cyst established by Evans called for assessment of the lesion in the aortoangiographic phase and the nephrographic phase by multiple tomograms. An avascular appearance of the mass and absence of abnormal perforating vessels during the aortoangiographic phase, homogeneous radiolucency and a sharp demarcation against normal functioning parenchyma during the nephrographic phase, demonstration of a well defined thin wall delineating the lesion and an acute sharp angle segment denoting the junction and demarcation of cyst and cortex are the original criteria advocated for the diagnosis of renal cysts (Table VII) (87) (Fig. 27). Bosniak and his co-workers stressed that a cyst should show a wall-thickness no greater than the line created by a very fine sharply pointed pencil (39). A thicker or irregular wall indicates the presence of a cystic or necrotic carcinoma. Bosniak attributed many errors in diagnosis to ignorance of this telltale characteristic of necrotic hypernephromas (Fig. 5) .

The necessity of fine detail demonstration emphasizes the need

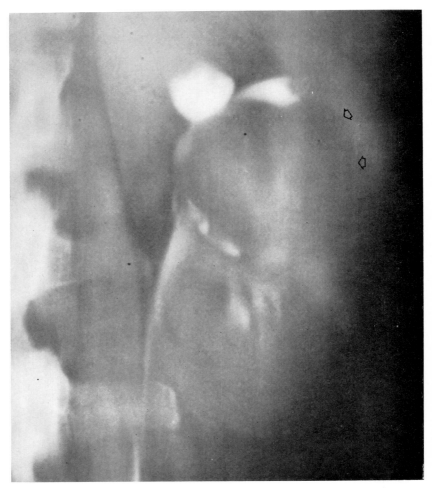

FIGURE 27. A nephrotomogram demonstrates a homogeneously radiolucent mass with sharp demarcation against normal functioning parenchyma. Splaying of the infundibula of the mid- and superior calyceal group is noted. There is evidence of a bulbous caliectasis of one of the calyces of the superior calyceal group, presumably secondary to obstruction by direct pressure from this cyst.

for high technical quality of nephrotomograms. The demonstration of a lesion on aortoangiographic and nephrographic phasetomograms necessitates several massive intravenous injections of contrast medium. Since several laminographic cuts should be obtained to properly outline the lesion on each phase, up to four rapid bolus injections of contrast medium are necessary to perform this study according to the technique described by Evans (87). A modified intravenous drip infusion technique provides a sustained nephrogram allowing ample time to obtain multiple sections through the entire kidney and possibly even repeat examination at the volition of the examiner (247) (Fig. 5). The aortoangiographic phase, however, cannot be depicted by this method. The drip infusion technique, in conjunction with laminography, is now the most commonly practiced form of nephrotomography because of its simplicity and propensity for a reproducible quality examination. Only a combination of a rapid sequence film changer with laminographic attachment permits demonstration of all essential phases on laminographic cuts with a single rapid bolus injection of contrast medium (126, 175, 218).

A wide range of accuracy has been reported for nephrotomographic diagnosis of renal mass lesions (54, 87, 88, 89, 90, 91, 163, 218, 287). Evans, in summarizing the series of Southwood and his own experience, found a percentage of error of 4 percent in normals, 5 percent in renal cysts, 6 percent in renal carcinoma, and 4 percent in miscellaneous entities (Table VIII) (91). Witten, who established a similar rate of accuracy for cysts or neoplasms, recorded indeterminate studies in approximately 3 percent of all patients in his series (287). The statistical significance of the indeterminate group has been stressed by many authors (39, 163, 218). A rate of accurate diagnosis of 95 percent can be expected only in those cases of renal cysts in which all characteristic nephrotomographic features can be demonstrated. Petersen asserted that, in his series of 103 cases, a clear cut pattern was appreciated in only one-half of the patients, the other one-half was relegated to the indeterminate group showing an equivocal radiolucent mass and pyelocalyceal deformity (218). Bosniak reported a similar experience in his large series of more than 500 nephrotomograms and attributed the overall accuracy rate of 75 percent to lack of accurate diagnosis in this indeterminate group. Our own experience confirms this impression and emphasizes the superiority of renal arteriography for the diagnosis of certain avascular renal carcinomas (Table IX). Five patients with nephrotomographic criteria suggesting a benign cyst were found to show abnormal vessels on selective renal arteriograms after adrenalin injection. Five other patients, likewise with nephrotomographic criteria of a benign cyst, demonstrated neovascularity in the rim of an avascular lesion on the renal arteriogram (Table IX). Two more patients with nephrotomographic criteria of a benign cyst were identified as renal tumors on the basis of collateral vessels or a tumor stain on selective renal arteriograms (Table IX). The erroneous diagnosis of a necrotic renal tumor was made in at least 8 patients on basis of nephrotomographic criteria. Seven of these patients were proven to have inflammatory lesions, one a benign cyst (Table IX) (Fig. 28). However, the selective renal arteriogram, similarly failed to identify many of the inflammatory lesions. The difficulty of properly identifying renal abscesses or inflammatory lesions by nephrotomography and selective renal angiography has been confirmed by other investigators (37).

Nephrotomography has been advocated as a simple screening technique for assessment of renal mass lesions, capable of delivering an accurate answer in about 75 percent of the patients thus examined. Drip infusion nephrotomography is particularly lauded for its ability to establish the presence or absence of a renal mass following inconclusive excretory urography and frequently obviates the necessity for more sophisticated procedures. The simplicity and safety of this technique advocates its use in the elderly arteriosclerotic patient. The possibility of utilizing this technique on an outpatient basis offers a distinct medico-economic advantage. Although usually not definitive by itself, nephrotomography if complemented by renal angiography and cyst puncture, aspiration and histopathologic assessment of the aspirant, offers optimal diagnostic accuracy for biologic techniques.

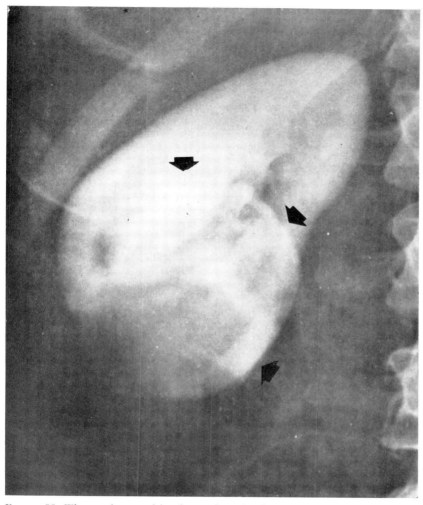

FIGURE 28. The nephrographic phase of a selective renal arteriogram demonstrates a radiolucent mass in the lower pole of the right kidney. The margins of this lesion, however, appear to show a homogeneously increased stain but lack abnormal vessels. A diagnosis of inflammatory cyst was made on basis of this observation and subsequently confirmed. Lack of neovascularity or abnormal vessels following the circumference of the lesion permits differentiation against a cystic and necrotic hypernephroma. (Courtesy, Lang — Journal of Urology.)

ANGIOGRAPHY OF RENAL CYSTS

The arteriographic characteristics of renal cysts are a spherical and crescentic displacement pattern of small and attenuated vessels around a nonstaining mass. There must not be demonstrable perforating vessels entering the mass, arteriovenous aneurysms, puddling of contrast medium or prominent draining veins (48). The capillary and nephrographic phases should demonstrate a sharp demarcation between cyst and adjacent normal parenchyma. Sharp margins and the demonstration of a subcapsular "spur" formed by normally staining parenchyma bordering the cyst are mandatory to affirm the diagnosis by arteriogram (Fig. 29, 30, 21).

The reliability of the renal angiogram for differentiation of poorly vascularized renal tumors and renal cysts has been questioned by some investigators (269). While this doubt in the diagnostic ability was justified for arteriographic assessment of renal cysts by translumbar aortography, selective renal arteriography and the concomitant use of pharmacologic agents such as epinephrine have vastly improved our ability to identify cystic and necrotic tumors. The diagnostic accuracy of selective angiography, however, is directly proportional to the technical quality of the examination, the appropriate utilization of pharmacologic agents accentuating tumor vessels and, particularly, the experience of the examiner (189, 212, 228). Certain solid tumors, deserve our particular attention because of the difficult differentiation against renal cysts by arteriography. Tubular and papillary adenocarcinomas have a very meager blood supply and, hence, demonstrate on arteriogram an interface between normal parenchyma and tumor that simulates a cyst (26). Certain metastatic carcinomas to the kidney are likewise extremely avascular and may, therefore, simulate a cyst. Infected cysts, conversely, demonstrate abnormal vessels in the wall of the cyst and may, mimic a necrotic and cystic hypernephroma on arteriograms (26, 185).

In our own experience, the arteriogram was proven reliable for the diagnosis of renal cysts. Of a total of 106 patients in this group, 102 benign simple cysts were accurately diagnosed by this modality (163) (Table VI). This accuracy rate of greater than 96 percent is acceptable in biological sciences. Nephrotomog-

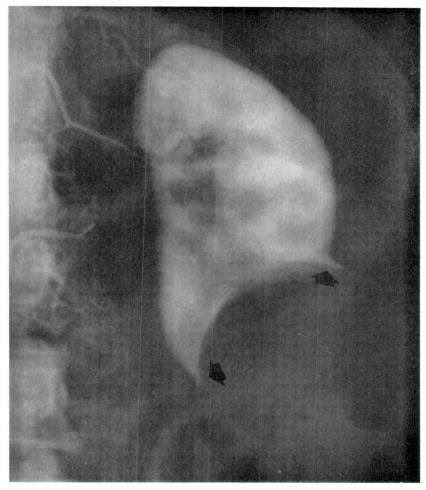

FIGURE 29. The nephrographic phase of a selective renal arteriogram demonstrates the characteristic interphase of parenchyma and cyst and a subcapsular "spur" formed by normally staining parenchyma bordering a subcapsular cyst (arrows).

raphy established a definitive and accurate diagnosis in only 79 percent of the patients with benign solitary renal cysts (Table VI). The lesion most commonly misdiagnosed as renal cyst was the renal adenoma. Eight renal adenomas of a total group of 41 examined by arteriogram were erroneously diagnosed as renal cysts (Table VI) (163).

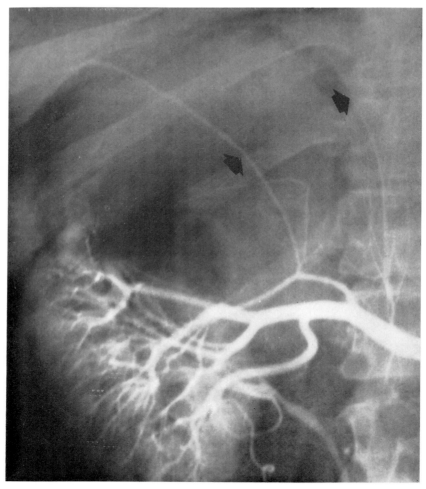

FIGURE 30. The arterial phase of a selective renal angiogram demonstrates a huge avascular mass in the upper pole of the right kidney. Note the characteristic splaying of the superior and midcapsular and midadrenal arteries *(arrows)*. A subcapsular "spur" along the lateral margin supports the diagnosis of a benign cyst. The study was combined with a retroperitoneal gas study to assess for dissectability of the mass against other retroperitoneal structures and to improve detail demonstration of small vessels.

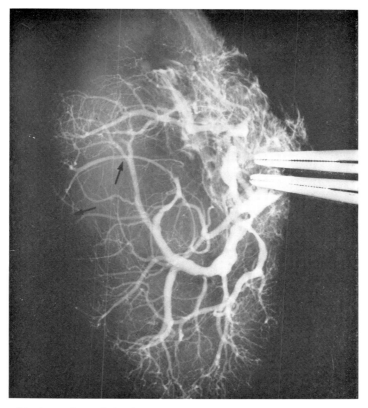

FIGURE 31. A specimen injection roentgenogram demonstrates the characteristic splaying of interlobar arteries around a small intrarenal cyst *(arrows)*.

The renal arteriogram may be able to diagnose a tumor within a cyst (48, 164). Although a definitive diagnosis of this combination was established on basis of the arteriogram in only 3 of 5 patients, the arteriogram greatly advanced our understanding of the pathophysiology of this lesion. The demonstration of abnormal vessels seemingly distributed over the circumference of a globe-like structure suggested that the tumor arose within the sheath of a renal cyst. The accuracy of this arteriographic demonstration was confirmed on the resected specimen in a patient who had been followed over a period of six years with multiple intravenous urograms with the diagnosis of renal cyst (164) (Table XIV) (Fig. 46a, b, c, d, e).

On the basis of the experience reported in the recent literature and our own series, arteriography appears capable of providing a reasonably accurate diagnosis of renal cysts. The false-positive diagnosis of lesions simulating renal cysts such as tubular or papillary adenocarcinomas, benign renal adenomas, metastatic carcinomas and, in rare instances, avascular hypernephromas, can be excluded by utilizing confirmatory examinations such as cyst puncture, aspiration and histochemical examination of the aspirant (158).

CYST PUNCTURE, ASPIRATION AND DOUBLE CONTRAST STUDY OF CYSTS

The continuing increase in our older age population, the predominant occurrence of asymptomatic renal mass lesions in patients past the fifth decade and the increased surgical risk in older patients or even contraindication of surgical exploration because of concurrent medical disease have created a growing pool of patients in whom the definitive diagnosis of renal cyst must be established on basis of nonoperative diagnostic studies (46, 77, 108, 144, 151, 168, 186, 209, 221, 223, 280). The accuracy rate achieved by the sum total of all diagnostic studies other than cyst puncture is in the 90 percent range for the diagnosis of renal cysts. This denotes the need for further and more definitive affirmation of the diagnosis. Cyst puncture, aspiration of fluid, histochemical and histopathological studies of the cyst content, and double contrast roentgenographic study of the cyst have been advocated to confirm the diagnosis and obviate surgical exploration. In the past, percutaneous cyst puncture and aspiration had been advocated primarily for confirmation of the clinical diagnosis of renal cyst in patients of the older age group or in patients with other medical disease mitigating against surgical exploration (68, 69, 108, 144, 216, 286). Increasing experience and, particularly, confirmation of the accuracy of this technique on basis of larger series, however, have expanded its application (23). Cyst puncture, aspiration and double contrast study is now advocated for substantiation of the diagnosis of renal cyst in all patients in whom other clinical or laboratory studies such as intravenous urography, retrograde urography, nephrotomography, arteriography, and histochemical studies of urine and blood have suggested the presence of a renal cyst and in whom there are no compelling reasons for surgical intervention (23, 46, 68, 69, 77, 108, 144, 154, 157, 158, 163, 164, 166, 285).

The battery of examinations combined with cyst puncture, aspiration and double contrast study defacto affords the patient an interdisciplinary approach to the problem. Cyst puncture per se is a form of surgical exploration of the mass lesion (63, 69). The histochemical examination of the aspirant permits a detailed biochemical assessment for metabolic by-products of tumor. The histopathological examination of the aspirants aided by cell block and Papanicolaou smears offers a detailed pathological assessment second only to serial sections of the removed specimen. The double contrast study allows appraisal of the cyst wall and demonstration of any possible mass lesion protruding into the lumen of the cyst (Fig. 32a, b, 33a, b, 34, 35a, b, c, 36). Laminography of the opacified cyst permits further detailed assessment of the cyst at various levels. Superimposition of laminograms of the opacified cavity upon the negative nephrotomographic filling defect, preferably in two planes, establishes with certainty whether the entire negative defect is explained on basis of the opacified cyst. This process serves to exclude any obscure neighboring mass lesion (69, 76, 77, 144).

The first pertinent observation is relevant to the cyst puncture and aspiration of fluid. Failure of fluid aspiration, "a dry tap," should be confirmed by ascertaining that the tip of the needle is in the center of the suspected mass lesion on roentgenograms obtained in right angle planes (63, 69, 76, 77, 144, 196, 216). A documented "dry tap" indicates the presence of a neoplasm or benign tumor. Whenever possible, exploration of such a lesion should follow as promptly as possible. In most instances, the presence of tumor was confirmed in lesions exhibiting the phenomenon of a "dry tap" (76, 108, 196, 216). Occasionally, exploration will merely reveal a simple solitary cyst which evaded detection by the probing needle

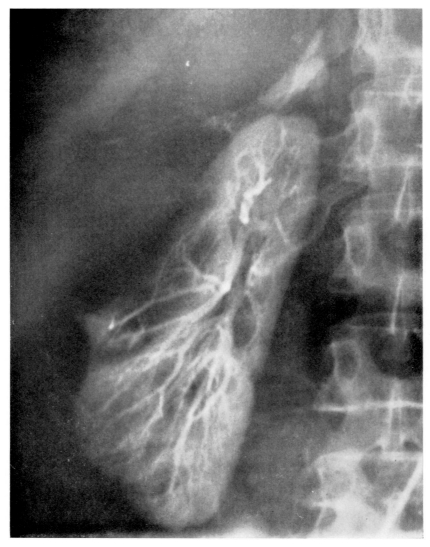

FIGURE 32a, b. A selective renal arteriogram suggests the presence of a large subcapsular cyst arising from the lateral circumference of the right kidney. Note the typical parenchymal "spur" *(arrow)*. A double contrast cyst study demonstrates a subcapsular cyst which appears to fit the depressed parenchymal components outlined on the preceding arteriogram.

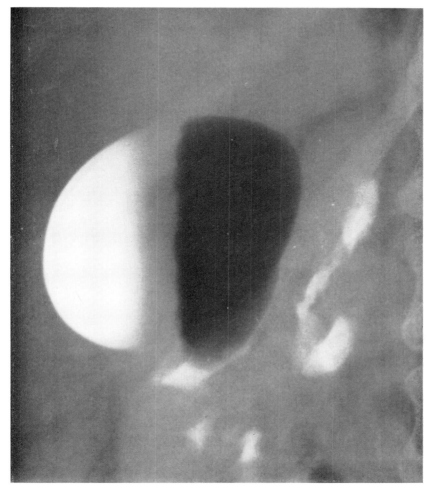

FIGURE 32b.

(286) . Although it is often difficult to prove this point, it is suspected that the tip of the needle might not have been placed within the lesion and that documentation of the needle position on AP
and crosstable lateral roentgenograms had not been obtained.

Aspiration of discolored or bloody fluid, likewise, raises the
question of a necrotic or cystic tumor (Table XIII) . Exceptions

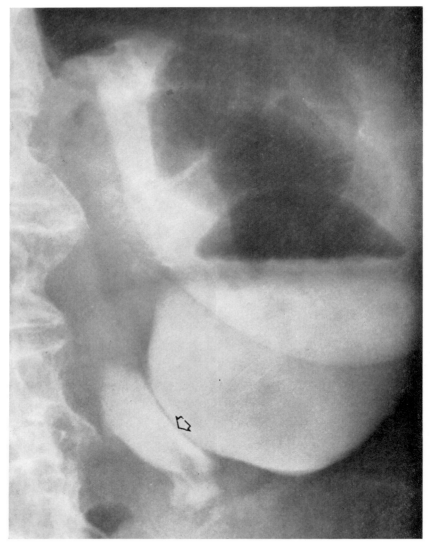

FIGURE 33a, b. A double contrast cyst study demonstrates a huge cyst arising from the upper pole of the left kidney which causes a slight tilt of the renal axis and compression of the pelvis. Upright and multiple decubitus positions demonstrate a smooth lining of the cyst. The aspiration of crystal clear yellowish fluid and histochemical and histopathological examination of the aspirant confirmed the diagnosis of a benign cyst.

to this rule, however, have been reported with increasing frequency (144, 154, 156, 163). In our own series, 11 of 129 patients with benign cysts showed either cloudy or bloody aspirant. The hemorrhagic content was explained, in most instances, on basis of a traumatic tap. Cloudy fluid may possibly reflect an ancient inflammatory process (Table XIII). A similar experience was reported by Kaiser, who found cloudy or bloody aspirant in 2 of 31 pa-

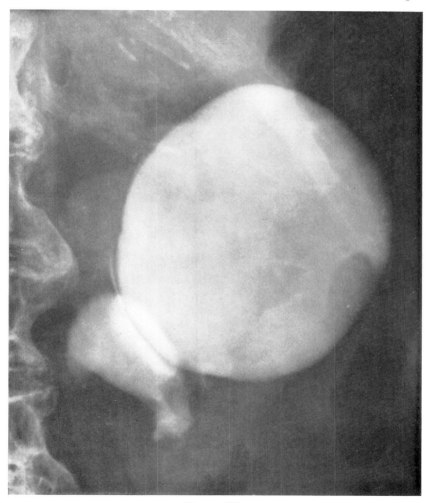

FIGURE 33b.

tients, both of whom demonstrated merely a serous cyst at exploration (144). Deweerd and Lalli proved the traumatic puncture concept by demonstrating abrasions in the far wall of the

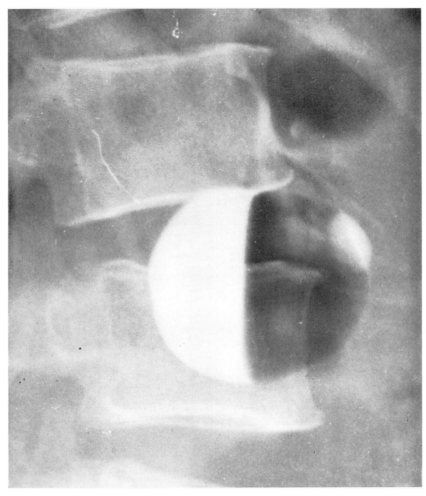

FIGURE 34a, b. A double contrast cyst study demonstrates two non-communicating cysts in the lower pole of the right kidney. The initial study showed a remaining unexplained spherical filling defect which, after subsequent direct puncture and injection with contrast medium, proved to be a second small neighbor cyst *(arrow)*.

cyst in a few instances on subsequent exploration of the lesion (69, 154).

While crystal-clear and yellowish aspirant has been advocated as a reliable criterion for the diagnosis of a benign cyst, occasional association of tumors with a cyst revealing such clear fluid has been reported (18, 148, 195, 231). However, the generalization

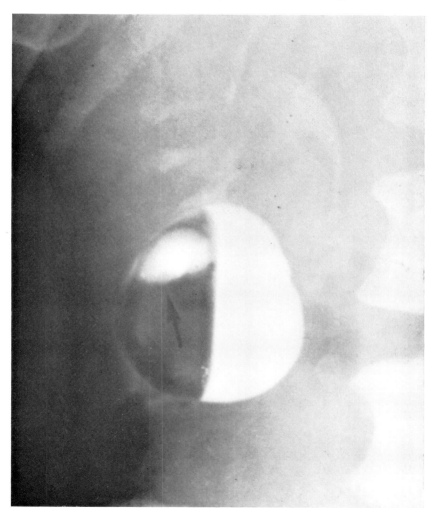

FIGURE 34b.

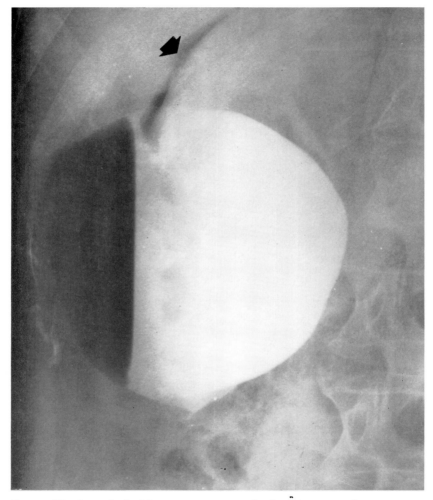

FIGURE 35a, b, c. A double contrast cyst study demonstrates a huge cyst occupying the lower pole of the right kidney. The lining of the cyst is delineated in multiple upright and decubitus positions and demonstrates a smooth surface. Note retroperitoneal gas dissection secondary to leakage of air through the puncture hole of the cyst.

that crystal-clear yellow aspirant indicates a benign cyst whereas discolored, cloudy or bloody aspirant favors a necrotic tumor or

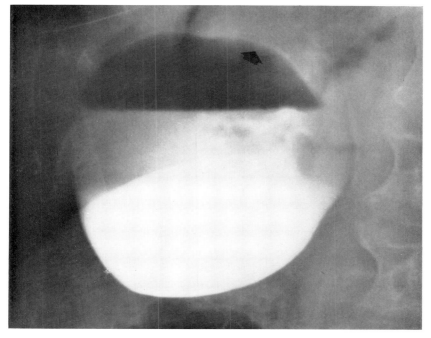

FIGURE 35b.

cyst associated with a tumor remains pertinent to our diagnostic thinking.

Histochemical examination of the aspirant has been introduced recently. Gernert analyzed the aspirant and found the pH to be usually alkaline, the specific gravity consistent with urine, urea nitrogen, glucose and chloride elevated as compared to the serum composition, while the total protein appeared to be extremely low (108). He noted that, in their series of 100 patients, no tumors were discovered within a cyst if clear and straw-colored fluid was aspirated and the chemical constituents were within normal range. Based on the concept that the fat content of fluid is markedly elevated if a shedding or necrotic tumor without epithelial lining is immersed, we have advocated examination of the aspirant for fat. In 122 of 132 patients with proven benign cysts, a Sudan III stain of the cyst fluid examined in a white cell cham-

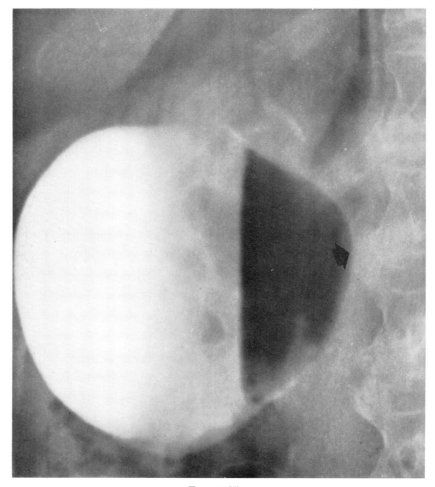

FIGURE 35c.

ber revealed no evidence of fat globules (Table XIII). In eight instances, a trace of fat was present, however, one of these patients was later proven to have an inflammatory cyst. In only two patients was the fat content high. Both of these patients proved to have an inflammatory cyst. Conversely, the fat content was high in all necrotic and cystic tumors and in 4 of 5 patients with a tumor associated with a cyst (Table XIII) (158, 163, 164). On the basis

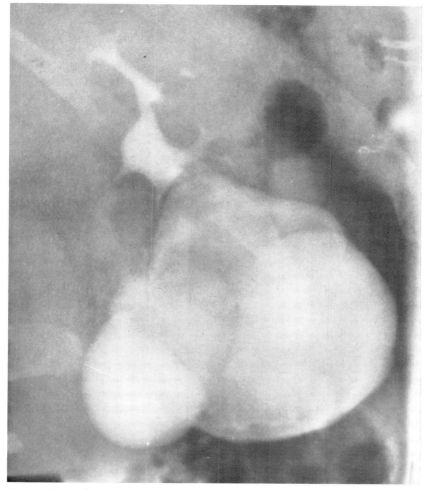

FIGURE 36. A double contrast cyst study demonstrates a compound multilocular cyst. Superimposition of the nephrotomogram demonstrating a multinodular avascular mass and the opacified cystogram showed perfect coincidence of the lesion.

of these statistical deliberations, much credence is attributed to fat content of aspirated cyst fluid as indicator of a benign cyst, associated inflammatory disease, or a necrotic tumor. Our experience suggests that an error margin of less than 2 percent would

TABLE+ XIII

THE CAPABILITY OF ACCURATE DIAGNOSIS OF VARIOUS TESTS PERFORMED IN CONJUNCTION WITH RENAL CYST PUNCTURE AND ASPIRATION

	Pathological Diagnosis	Correct Pre-op Diagnosis	Correct Roentgeno-graphic Diagnosis	Fat			Fluid			Pap.		
				None	Trace	High	Clear	Cloudy	Bloody	−	?	+
Cysts*	129	124	124	122	7	—	118	2	9	108	21	—
Tumor in Cyst	5	5	5	—	1	4	—	2	3	—	1	4
Necrotic Tumors**	17	17	16	—	—	16	—	4	12	—	—	17**
Inflammatory Cysts	3	3	3	—	1	2	—	2	1	1	2	—

*Parapelvic multilocular and solitary.
**Dry tap (aspiration—cell block).
+Courtesy, Lang—Journal of Urology.

result if the diagnosis of benign cystic disease were based on the observation that the aspirated cyst fluid contained no or only a trace of fat (Table XIII).

Following the suggestion of Gernert, we are now assessing cyst fluid for protein content and find aspirant from benign cysts to show an extremely low protein content whereas fluid aspirated from necrotic tumors shows a remarkably high protein content.

Histopathologic assessment of aspirated fluid has been advocated only in the recent past (144, 158). Although statistical data are not available from the literature, it is inferred that Papanicolaou smears on cell blocks of cyst aspirant would render a 100 percent accurate diagnosis. While, in our experience, the Papanicolaou smear was 100 percent accurate in the diagnosis of all necrotic tumors and in the majority of tumors within a cyst or cyst wall, a significant number of indeterminate PAP grades were assigned to fluid aspirated from benign cysts, parapelvic cysts, multilocular cysts and, particularly, inflammatory cysts (158, 163, 164, 166). A negative Papanicolaou reading was reported in about 84 percent of all benign cysts. Indeterminate Papanicolaou grades were reported in the remainder; none of the aspirants were classified as a positive Papanicolaou smear (Table XIII). On basis of our experience, it appears that credence can be attributed to both negative and positive readings of Papanicolaou smears whereas the indeterminate grade may indicate benign cysts, inflammatory cysts and, rarely, tumors associated with a cyst.

A double contrast study of a cyst is performed by replacing the aspirant with an equal amount of positive contrast medium and air (158). Appropriate positioning in upright, Trendelenburg and decubitus positions permits assessment of all perimeters of the cyst walls. While benign cysts will usually demonstrate a smooth spherical configuration, polyarcuate contour lines are also consistent with the diagnosis of benign cysts (154, 176, 177). Conformity of the lesion demonstrated on double contrast study to the negative defect seen on arteriograms or nephrotomograms in both AP and lateral projection roentgenograms is mandatory for an all inclusive diagnosis (69, 108, 154, 158, 176, 177, 285, 286). If one finds an unaccounted for component of the mass lesions after appropriate superimposition of cyst contrast studies and nephro-tomograms, further attempts must be directed to puncture the remaining unexplained space-occupying lesion. Only if the entire mass lesion is adequately explained, and the diagnosis of a cyst is assured may further diagnostic efforts cease (158, 163).

The demonstration of a mass lesion projecting into the lumen of the cyst is considered diagnostic for a tumor associated with a cyst (Fig. 48a, b, c) (Table XIV). In our series, a mass lesion was demonstrated in 4 of 5 patients with a proven coexistence of cyst and tumor. It should be stressed that such a tumor may be benign or malignant. Recent reports of benign intracystic fibromas and leiomyomas presenting as polypoid tumors within a cyst have confirmed the coexistence of cysts and benign tumors (60, 188). Occasionally, a mass lesion in an opacified cyst has been simulated on laminograms by the polyarcuate components of a cyst wall pro-truding into the lumen (144). A differentiation of a protruding cyst component and a tumor however, should be possible by dem-onstrating the smooth surface and continuity of such a polyarcu-ate structure with the cyst wall on different projections. A tumor arising from the lining of the cyst wall, need not necessarily im-part the appearance of a true mass lesion projecting into the lumen of the cyst. In one of our patients, the tumor was limited to the cyst wall and failed to produce a demonstrable mass within the lumen of the cyst (Fig. 46a, b, c, d, e) (Table XIV). This lesion, however, was readily diagnosable on basis of the character-istic arteriographic findings and the telltale findings of the histo-chemical and histopathological examination of the aspirant. (164). Brannan described a similar finding on a pathological specimen and it is suspected that had a cyst puncture and double contrast study been performed, this lesion would likewise have failed to demonstrate protrusion of tumor into the lumen.

A statistical evaluation of the diagnostic accuracy of roentgeno-graphic double contrast studies of renal cysts and necrotic and cystic tumors reveals an accuracy of 96 percent (Table XIII). Combining the roentgenographic findings with the laboratory examination of the aspirant, the correct diagnosis was established in 149 patients of a total group of 154 although a somewhat lower diagnostic confidence level had to be assigned to 9 of the patients because of disparity of the various diagnostic indices Table XIII) .

PERI- AND PARAPELVIC CYSTS

Parapelvic cysts are thin-walled structures that may or may not communicate with the renal pelvis or calyces (2, 15, 31, 32, 94, 105, 119, 251, 270) . Noncommunicating parapelvic cysts contain a straw-colored fluid and may be of variable size, single or multiple.

Peri- and parapelvic cysts are relatively uncommon (15) . A nephrotomographic survey of renal mass lesions reveals that parapelvic cysts account for only about 4 percent of all renal cysts (73) . Williams established an incidence rate of 0.15 percent of this condition in the general urologic patient population (282) .

The etiology of peri- and parapelvic cysts remains a matter of considerable controversy (2, 15, 31, 32, 73, 198, 208, 262) . It has been suggested that parapelvic cysts developed from congenital Wolffian bodies or mesonephric rests (2, 249) . This theory, however, has not gained many supporters. Henthorne suggested that these cysts are of lymphatic origin and probably the result of chronic inflammation causing lymphangiectasia (70, 129, 182) . In addition to these etiologic factors, there is convincing evidence that some parapelvic cysts may result as late sequelae to conservative management of closed renal injury (132, 137, 166) . Several well documented cases have shown development of a parapelvic cyst following blunt or penetrating renal trauma (132, 256) .

The roentgenographic findings of a noncommunicating parapelvic cyst on a flat plate of the abdomen merely indicate the presence of a perihilar soft tissue mass which may sometimes blurr the psoas shadow (105) . The intravenous urograms may show compression and displacement of the renal pelvis and calyces and elongation of the infundibula. Because of the hilar origin, an expanding cyst may displace the normal perihilar fat causing a crescentic radiolucent shadow enveloping the periphery of this perihilar mass (251) . Since noncommunicating parapelvic cysts are defacto extrarenal and not surrounded by renal parenchyma,

TABLE XIV*
DIAGNOSTIC ABILITY OF VARIOUS PROCEDURES FOR
IDENTIFICATION OF TUMORS IN CYST

	Positive Diagnosis
Total No.	5
KUB	0
IVP	0
Nephrotomogram	0
Scintiscan	0
Arteriogram	3
Positive Double	
Control Cyst Study	5
Fat none	—
Fat low	1
Fat high	4
Pap Smear +Cell Block —	—
Pap Smear +Cell Block ?	1
Pap Smear +Cell Block +	4
Fluid clear	—
Fluid cloudy	2
Fluid bloody	3

ASPIRANT ANALYSIS

*Courtesy, Lang, E.K.—Journal of Urology.

there is no sharply defined demarcation against the opacified renal parenchyma on the nephrographic phase roentgenograms (61).

Communicating peri- or parapelvic cysts present with an entirely different appearance on intravenous or retrograde pyelograms (15, 94, 119, 270). If the communication occurs through the calyx, as in the majority of the cases, the diagnosis can be made on basis of the diverticulum-like structure within the renal parenchyma (282). If the communication, however, extends through the wall of the renal pelvis, it may be difficult to distinguish such a lesion from hydronephrosis of the renal pelvis secondary to an aberrant blood vessel. Uson suggests the slow but progressive opacification of this "round cavity" with a propensity to retain the contrast medium after the pyelocalyceal system had emptied as reliable criteria for differentiation against hydronephrosis (Fig. 37a, b, c, d). A noteworthy absence of caliectasia and normal appearance of contrast medium in the pyelocalyceal system as well as a normal

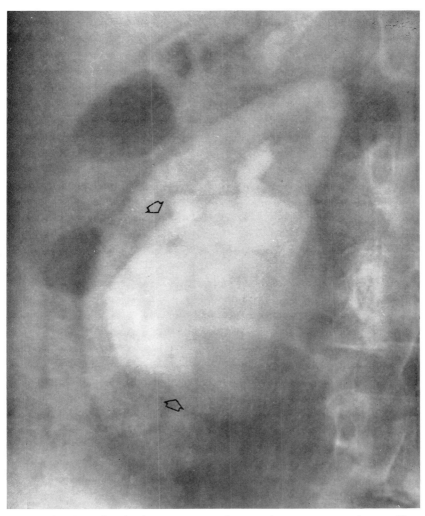

FIGURE 37a, b, c, d. The intravenous pyelogram demonstrates early opacification of normal appearing calyces and infundibula and delayed opacification of a "round cavity" which appears to communicate with the pelvis. A retrograde pyelogram demonstrates dense and early opacification of the cavity communicating with the pelvis. A delayed drainage film shows retention of contrast medium in the cavity.

Injection of contrast medium into one of the minor calyces by selective puncture demonstrated flow from the calyx into the pelvis without immediate opacification of this large communicating parapelvic cyst. The nature of a communicating parapelvic cyst is disclosed by selective puncture and injection of either the pyelocalyceal system or the communicating parapelvic cyst.

(Courtesy, Lang — Radiology.)

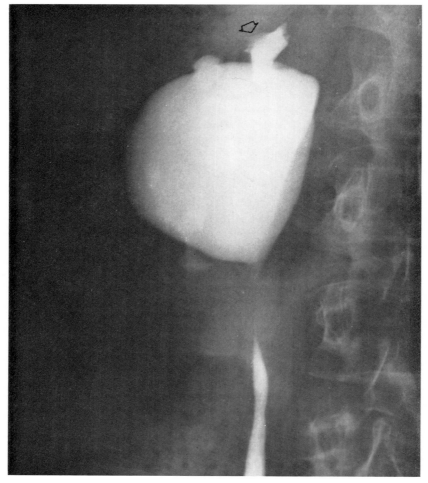

FIGURE 37b.

origin of the ureter from the ureteropelvic junction are other criteria useful for differentiation against hydronephrosis (270). However, large parapelvic cysts may not only obstruct the uretero-pelvic junction but can also cause progressive caliectasia and delayed dye excretion, hence a picture indistinguishable from that of a hydronephrosis. Williams thought that an inflammatory process caused formation of these cysts (282) (Fig. 38a, b). The possibility of

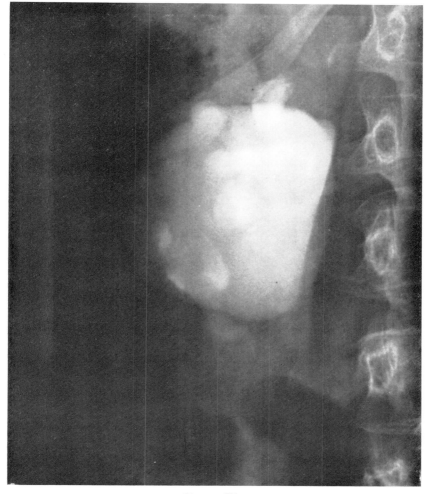

FIGURE 37c.

rupture of a cortical cyst into the calyceal system secondary to trauma cannot be excluded, however, this etiology is felt to contribute numerically very minimally to the development of such parapelvic or communicating cysts or diverticula (230).

Because of the lack of apposition to renal parenchyma, nephrotomography is only of limited use in the diagnosis of this entity.

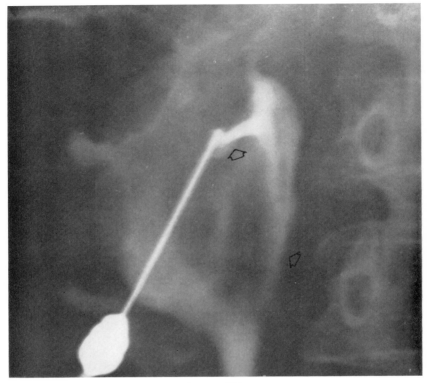

FIGURE 37d.

Selective renal arteriography, however, may provide findings diagnostic for a parapelvic cyst (55, 166). Splaying and displacement of the renal artery, but particularly the characteristic spherical displacement of the small pelvic branch vessels as well as the mid and inferior capsular artery, are the diagnostic hallmarks of this entity (Fig. 39a, b). Nephrographic phase roentgenograms demonstrate characteristic lateral displacement of the parenchyma with minimal effacement by the parapelvic mass. Unlike most other medial space-occupying lesions, parapelvic cysts will usually not result in change of the kidney axis but merely displace the kidney laterally. Absence of abnormal vessels, a tumor strain, or puddling or pooling of contrast medium differentiate parapelvic cysts from hypernephromas that may have arisen near or extended

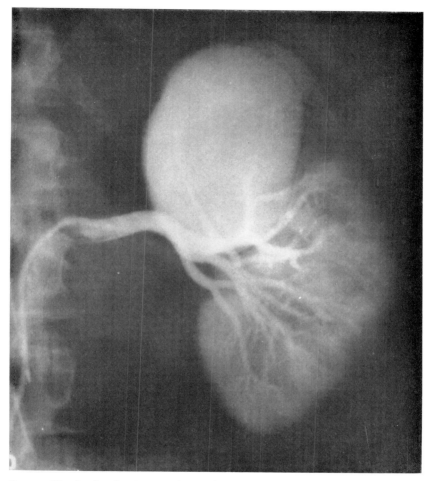

FIGURE 38a, b. A selective renal arteriogram demonstrates splaying and displacement of predominantly interlobar vessels around a partially intrarenal parapelvic cyst. A direct cyst puncture was carried out and the opacified cavity corresponded to the defect seen on the late phase arteriograms. The dye drainage from this cavity was delayed, however, a four-hour delayed film demonstrated that the cyst had emptied largely. The cyst was also demonstrable by retrograde intravenous pyelography. Exploration failed to show a definitive communication to the pyelocalyceal system and it was postulated that the communicating tract had sealed by recent inflammatory reaction. (Courtesy, Lang — Radiology.)

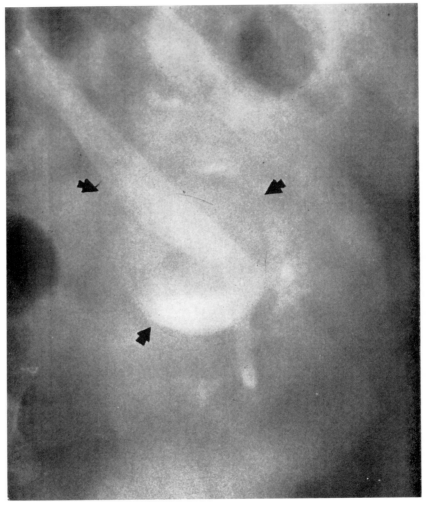

FIGURE 38b.

into the renal pelvis or propagated to the parapelvic area via the renal vein (Fig. 40a, b, c, 41a, b). Other vascular tumors involving the hilum of the kidney are distinguishable from parapelvic cysts on basis of characteristic arteriographic stain (120).

Cyst puncture, aspiration, histochemical and histopathological examination of the aspirant, and double contrast studies of the cyst have served to affirm the diagnosis. In 5 of 6 patients of our

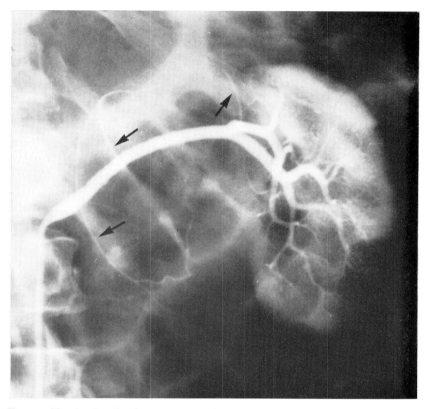

FIGURE 39a, b. A selective renal arteriogram demonstrates marked displacement and splaying of the main renal artery over and around a spherical mass which displaces the kidney laterally. Note the characteristic splaying and spherical configuration of the capsular and pelvic branch vessels identifying this lesion as a parapelvic cyst. Lack of a stain of abnormal vessels in the area of the described mass lesion on late phase roentgenograms differentiates parapelvic cysts against central hypernephromas. (Courtesy, Lang — Radiology.)

series, a spherical cyst encroaching upon the renal pelvis could be demonstrated by double contrast study of the cysts (Table VI). The sixth patient showed that the opacified cyst had completely emptied on a four-hour delayed film and hence confirmed the presence of communication to the pyelocalyceal system. The precise communication, however, could not be demonstrated roent-

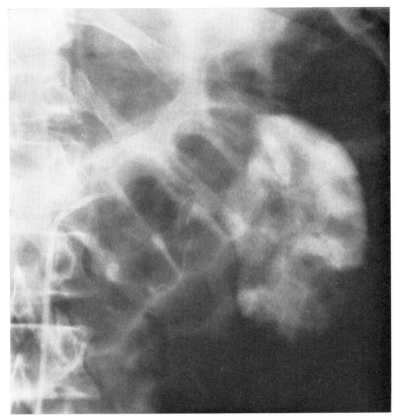

FIGURE 39b.

genographically (22) (Fig. 38a, b) . The validity of this observation on the double contrast cyst study was confirmed by retrograde pyelography. After an initial delay, there was sudden opacification of the parapelvic cyst, however, again oblique and lateral
projections failed to demonstrate the communication to the pelvis. On this occasion, the parapelvic cyst remained opacified for
two days although progressive decrease of dye density was observed on serial roentgenograms. On the third day, the patient ex-
perienced increasing back pain and demonstrated a marked
febrile reaction. During exploration and marsupialization of the

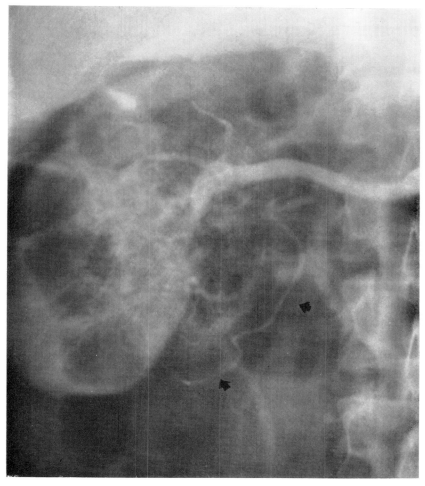

FIGURE 40a, b, c. A selective renal arteriogram pre-empted by an injection of adrenalin hydrochloride demonstrates a staining mass in the perihilar area of the right kidney. The observation of abnormal corkscrew vessels and puddling of dye identifies the lesion as a hypernephroma. The lesion occasions a similar displacement pattern of the mid-capsular artery *(arrows)* as parapelvic cysts. (Courtesy, Lang — Radiology.)

cyst, we could not identify a definite communication from the cyst to the pyelocalyceal system, however, evidence of recent inflam-

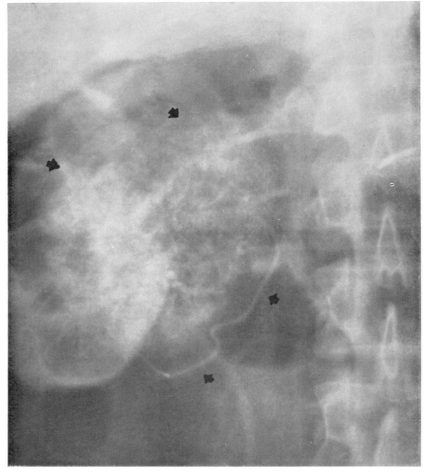

FIGURE 40b.

matory reaction was noted and it was postulated that the communicating tract might have sealed (59) (Fig. 38a, b).

Two of our patients with parapelvic cysts deserve special attention because of a history suggesting a traumatic etiology. A classical noncommunicating parapelvic cyst was demonstrated in one patient in whom a calculus had been removed through the renal pelvis some eighteen years earlier. Intravenous urograms ob-

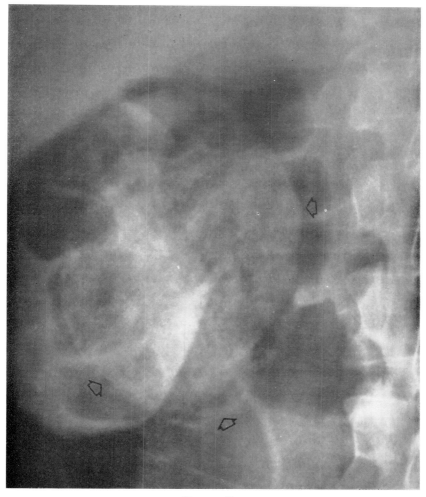

FIGURE 40c.

tained prior to the surgical procedure failed to demonstrate the presence of a parapelvic cyst. The urographic, arteriographic, and double contrast studies of this parapelvic cyst were indistinguishable from parapelvic cysts of noncommunicating type of other etiology. In one other patient, an even more convincing demonstration was rendered. A communicating type of parapelvic cyst was

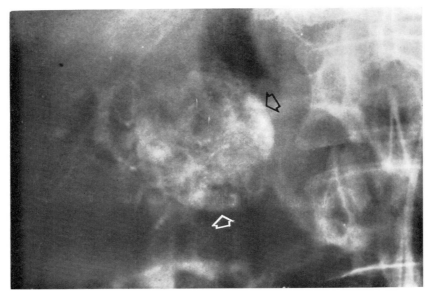

FIGURE 41a, b. A selective renal arteriogram of the right kidney preluded by an injection of adrenalin hydrochloride demonstrates a cluster of abnormal vessels. The abnormal staining mass occupies the perihilar area similar to a parapelvic cyst but is readily differentiated on basis of abnormal vessels and sustained tumor stain *(arrows)*. (Proven hypernephroma.)

demonstrated some eight months after severe blunt renal trauma. An arteriogram performed on the day of the blunt renal trauma had shown subcapsular severance of renal parenchyma of the midportion of the kidney. The nephrographic phase roentgenogram demonstrated a 2 cm wide segment of adjacent parenchyma exhibiting markedly decreased parenchymal stain presumably secondary to traumatic thrombosis of the smaller vessels. Although hematuria persisted for nine days, conservative management was persued. Intravenous urograms obtained at weekly intervals failed to show any abnormality for the first month. However, an intravenous urogram obtained at a follow-up visit some eight months later showed a typical communicating parapelvic cyst. The parapelvic cyst extended into the renal parenchyma in the region of the previously noted parenchymal tear (166) .

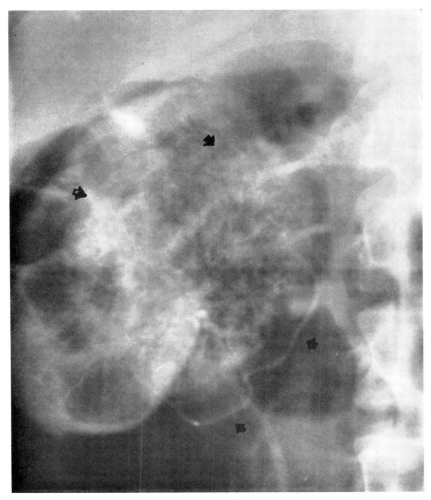

FIGURE 41b.

In our experience, a definitive diagnosis of parapelvic cyst was readily confirmed by cyst puncture, aspiration and double contrast study of the cyst. Arteriography demonstrated a characteristic displacement pattern of the renal artery and particularly of the pelvic and capsular branches and aided in excluding vascular tumors of the renal pelvis. Nephrotomography is of use only if the parapelvic cyst extends into the renal parenchyma and, hence, permits demonstration of an interface between normal renal parenchyma and a cyst. The retrograde pyelogram is advocated for assessment of any possible communication between the cyst and the pelvis or calyces. The intravenous urogram, while usually not diagnostic, may suggest the presence of a communicating para-pelvic cyst on basis of delayed contrast medium appearance in the cyst and markedly delayed emptying of contrast medium from the cyst exhibiting apparently normal calyceal structures. Noncom-municating parapelvic cysts may demonstrate pressure effect against the pelvis, infundibula and calyces. The demonstration of an ill defined soft tissue mass in the region of the pelvis causing dis-placement of the fat enveloping the renal pelvis merely suggests the presence of a space-occupying lesion originating from the renal pelvis. A differentiation of the type of space-occupying le-sion on the KUB is not possible and we have seen an identical pat-tern in at least one hypernephroma that extended directly into the renal pelvis (165, 166) (Fig. 41a, b).

MULTICYSTIC DISEASE

Multicystic disease is a rare entity attributed to a congenital fetal maldevelopment (56) (Table XII). Grossly, the kidney is re-placed by a cluster of cysts of varying size. The cysts are held to-gether by connective tissue, however, normal renal parenchyma is absent. The ureter is either absent or severely atrophic. Histologi-cally, there is a complete loss of renal architecture. Only occasion-ally a nubbin of solid tissue may be found which resembles infantile tubules or glomeruli. This suggests the embryologic de-fect to be a failure of union between the ureteral bud and the mesonephric blastema (83).

The intravenous urogram usually fails to show function be-cause of inability to concentrate contrast medium. This is in marked contradistinction to polycystic disease of the kidney which demonstrates distorted pyelocalyceal structures and compressed parenchyma on the roentgenograms depicting the nephrographic phase (56).

POLYCYSTIC DISEASE

Polycystic disease is of congenital origin with definitive hereditary tendencies and progressive in nature. Although unilateral polycystic disease of the kidney has been described, the common form is bilateral.

In contrast to the multicystic kidney, the polycystic kidney retains the renal contour and pyelocalyceal pattern though distorted by the cysts. Cysts vary greatly in size and in the adult form may reach enormous proportions. Histologically, the disease is characterized by normal-appearing nephrons interspersed among innumerable cysts. Irreversible progression of the disease is caused by continuous enlargement of the cysts with a resulting compression and destruction of the remaining normal renal parenchyma (83, 86).

The flat plate of the abdomen will usually demonstrate a large kidney with an irregular contour. The intravenous urogram is characterized by marked elongation of infundibula and splaying and displacement of calyces. Bulbous enlargement of the calyces is often observed in contrast to the narrowing, tapering, and destruction of the calyces occurring with neoplasm. A crescentic outline of the calyces due to pressure by an adjacent cyst is, likewise, a frequent finding. Distortion of the pelvis is only seldom encountered. The deformity usually involves all calyces, although findings may be accentuated in one part of the kidney. The retrograde pyelogram usually provides a better visualization, particularly in advanced disease with reduced renal function and a resulting poor excretory urogram.

The confirmation of polycystic disease of the kidney can be readily obtained on nephrotomograms. A characteristic "Swiss cheese" appearance best appreciated on the nephrographic phase establishes this diagnosis with great accuracy. Selective renal angiography has been advocated for differentiation of polycystic disease of the kidney and neoplastic entities. The renal arteriogram has been lauded for providing a clear assessment of the status of residual renal parenchyma. The classical appearance is that of stretching and splaying of renal arteries commensurate with the degree of involvement (Fig. 42a, b, 43a, b). There is, however, no

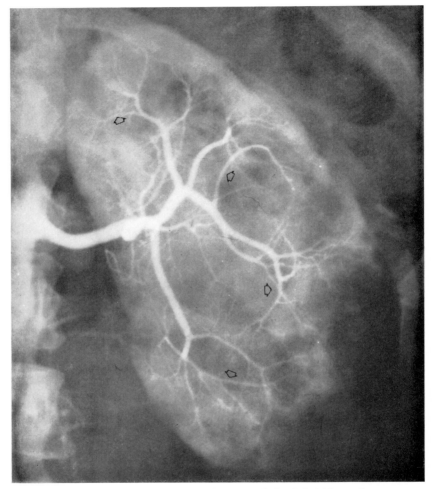

FIGURE 42a, b. A selective renal arteriogram of the left kidney demonstrates characteristic stretching and splaying of many interlobar arteries. There is no significant attenuation of the vessels. A delayed nephrographic phase film confirms the diagnosis of polycystic disease on basis of the characteristic "Swiss cheese" appearance.

significant tapering of the small renal branch arteries. Occasionally, impairment of flow through a renal vessel may result from a rapidly enlarging cyst (164, 166). The nephrographic phase of the selec-

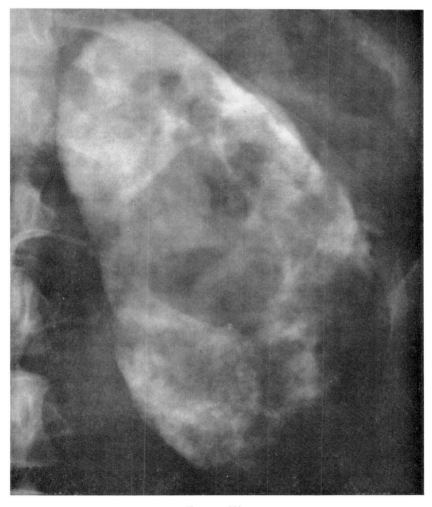

FIGURE 42b.

tive renal arteriogram permits assessment of the residual functioning parenchyma. A sustained nephrographic stain of some segments of renal parenchyma may indicate compression of the venous drainage by enlarging cysts and, hence, embarrassment of the
venous return (163) (Fig. 44a, b). It is postulated that the

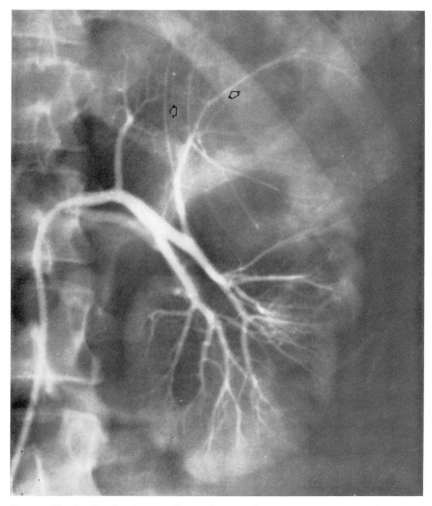

FIGURE 43a, b. A selective renal arteriogram demonstrates an essentially normal intrarenal vascular pattern in the lower one-half of the left kidney. Marked stretching and splaying of the interlobar arteries is noted in the upper one-half of the left kidney. A late phase roentgenogram demonstrates characteristic radiolucent cysts. In contrast to polycystic disease, this entity is characterized by involvement of only a portion of a kidney by multiple cysts of varying size. The prognosis appears to be better than that of genuine polycystic disease. (Courtesy, Lang — Radiology.)

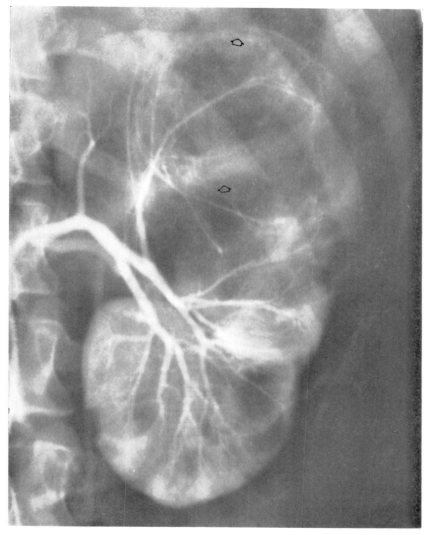

FIGURE 43b.

occurrence of hypertension in polycystic disease is not infrequently related to embarrassment of the vascular system by compression
of enlarging neighboring cysts (86).

Selective renal angiography is also of primary importance for the demonstration of renal cell carcinomas arising in a polycystic

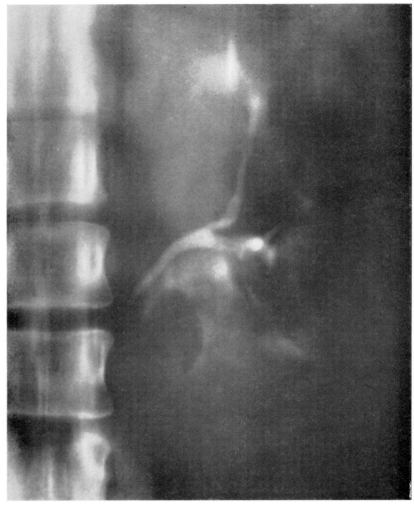

Figure 44a, b. A selective renal arteriogram demonstrates the classic displacement pattern of the interlobar arteries and the "Swiss cheese" appearance on the nephrographic phase tomograms. A selective injection of lower polar vessels shows an area of sustained nephrographic stain of renal parenchyma compressed by two enlarging cysts. The finding indicates embarrassment of venous return. (Courtesy, Lang — Radiology.)

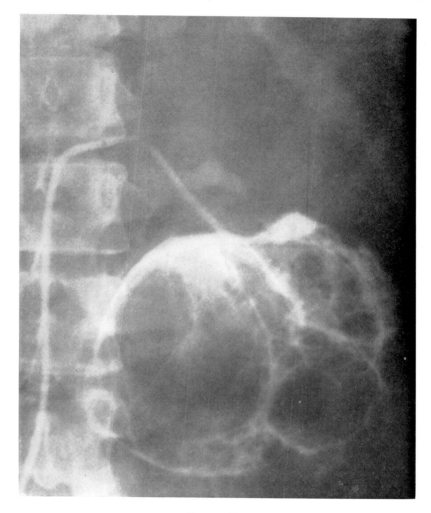

FIGURE 44b.

kidney. While this is not a common occurrence, it is by no means as infrequent as once thought. At least 19 cases of carcinoma arising in polycystic kidneys have been reported (42, 125, 134, 139, 164, 195). Abnormal vessels demonstrable in the residual parenchyma, subject to pressure by adjacent cysts and therefore arranged in a dome-shaped distribution pattern, are the characteristic arteriographic finding. A lack of responnse of these tumor vessels to epinephrine is considered diagnostic for renal cell carcinoma (3).

Scintiscanograms are likewise capable of identifying polycystic disease of the kidney on the basis of a characteristic "Swiss cheese appearance" of the scintiscanogram.

Cyst puncture, aspiration and double contrast studies are no longer advocated for diagnosis of this entity. In the past, this was proposed as the procedure of choice since it lent itself to decompression of a rapidly enlarging cyst (67). In some instances, sclerosing agents had been introduced hoping to cause permanent collapse and occlusion of the cyst. While a single cyst can be managed in this fashion, the procedure has no influence on the overall progression of the disease process and is, therefore, not capable of giving even temporary relief (63, 67).

CHAPTER IV

COEXISTENCE OF RENAL CYSTS AND CARCINOMA

T HE INCIDENCE RATE OF coexistent renal cyst and carcinoma greatly influences the decision of surgical versus conservative management of renal cysts. Coexistence of renal cysts and carcinoma in the same kidney has been reported as high as 30 percent and as low as 0.06 percent by various investigators (91, 281). Brannan, in a series of 104 renal cysts, found 4 carcinomas in cysts or involving the cyst wall (42). Emmett, reported coexistence of cyst and tumor in 10 patients in his large series of 438 patients with renal cysts (82). Kaiser, in a carefully worked-up series of 48 renal cysts, encountered only one cyst contiguous with a renal cell carcinoma (144). Lalli found 5 renal cell carcinomas associated with cysts in his series of 32 cysts (154). Coexistence of carcinoma and solitary renal cysts or parapelvic cysts has been reported by many other authors, however, an incidence rate of this occurrence was not established (148, 200, 215, 231, 235, 238, 241, 274, 276). A review of our pathological files revealed coexistence of cyst and tumor in 7 patients in a total series of 342 patients with proven renal cysts. This, again, establishes an incidence rate of approximately 2 percent. However, an assessment of coexistence of cyst and tumor in the same kidney in our series of 141 patients with various cysts evaluated by a complete modern diagnostic work-up disclosed 5 cases of this entity, an incidence rate of better than $3\frac{1}{2}$ percent (Table VI) (163, 164). We feel that this probably represents a realistic estimate of the occurrence rate of coexistent renal cyst and tumor.

Although clinically of subordinate importance, the coexistence of cysts and benign tumors has focused attention because of the difficulty of differentiating a benign tumor from a malignant one if occurring within a cyst (60, 188, 206, 245). Fortunately, these are rare lesions limited, in essence, to cystic hamartomas and cystadenomas (188, 227).

The relative frequency of coexistent cyst and tumor in one kidney emphasizes the necessity for complete evaluation by nephrotomography, selective renal angiography aided by pharmacologic agents, and cyst puncture, aspiration and double contrast study of cysts.

The ability of these studies to differentiate between renal cyst and tumor depends to a degree on the geographic relationship of cyst and tumor coexistent in the same kidney. Gibson established four possible relationships of cyst and tumor occurring in the same kidney: 1. widely separated lesions of unrelated origin; a chance occurrence, 2. origin of a cyst within a tumor; 3. origin of a tumor within a cyst, and 4. occurrence of a cyst distal to the tumor (110).

The accidental association of a serous renal cyst and a clear cell carcinoma in the same kidney is usually identifiable on nephrotomograms and selective renal angiograms. The confirmation of the benign nature of the serous cyst relies on cyst puncture, aspiration and double contrast study of the cyst. Histochemical and histopathological examination of the aspirant affirm the diagnosis. Laminography of the opacified cyst is useful to exclude the presence of small mass lesions protruding into the lumen of the cyst (54, 88, 91, 144, 158, 163).

Nephrotomography and selective renal angiography are the most important diagnostic modalities for establishing the diagnosis of a cystic and necrotic renal carcinoma. The demonstration of irregular and thick walls delineating such a lesion on nephrotomograms is highly suggestive of the diagnosis of cystic and necrotic hypernephroma (37) (Fig. 5). Inflammatory cysts, however, may mimic this nephrotomographic appearance and may even show increased vascularity on the aortoangiographic phase of the nephrotomograms (37) (Fig. 5). The demonstration of vessels of varying caliber accompanying and supplying such a mass by perpendicular, perforating branches has been considered diagnostic for a necrotic renal cell carcinoma (228). The lack of physiologic response of tumor vessels to adrenalin or epinephrine has been utilized to accentuate these relatively sparse tumor vessels in necrotic and cystic renal tumors (3, 140, 164). In many instances, the diagnosis of a cystic and necrotic tumor will hinge on the arteriographic demonstration of abnormal vessels accentuated by pharmacologic agents (Fig. 46a, b, c, d, e).

The angiographic pattern of a cystadenoma may be similar to

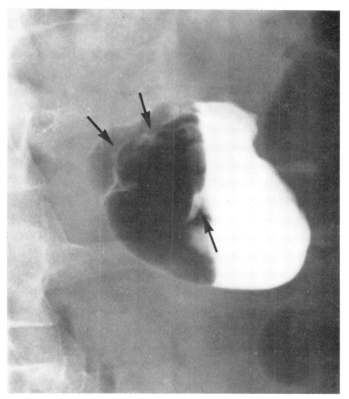

FIGURE 45a, b. A multilocular cyst is demonstrated on a double contrast cyst study in the lower pole of the left kidney. Several punctures were carried out to effect filling of all cysts, in particular several of the medial superior cyst group. Superimposition of the cystogram upon the nephrotomogram after the original puncture demonstrated a central filling defect that was not accounted for by the opacified cyst. Hence, repeated attempts at puncture were undertaken an ultimately delineated the presence of other centrally located cysts. (Courtesy, Lang — Journal of Urology.)

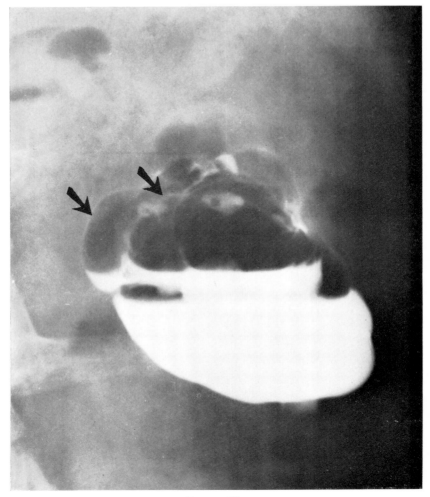

FIGURE 45b.

that of a malignant renal tumor (194, 234). Percutaneous cyst puncture, aspiration, histochemical and histopathological examination of the aspirant and double contrast study of the cyst is often unable to differentiate a benign tumor in a cyst from a malignant one (144, 188). McQueeney aspirated 30 cc of fluid from a cyst and demonstrated an intraluminal mass which was

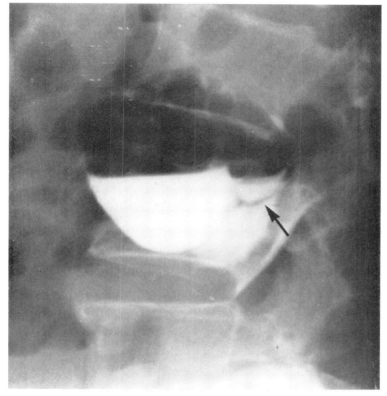

FIGURE 45c.

later proven to be an angiomyolipoma (188). Melicow reported a similar experience with a papillary cyst adenoma emphasizing the difficulty of establishing a preoperative diagnosis of such benign lesions (195).

Tumors arising within a cyst probably represent the rarest of these lesions and may cause some difficulty in diagnosis. It has been suggested in the literature that such tumors are not recognizable by selective renal angiography and that assessment of the aspirated fluid as to color and clarity did not provide reliable criteria (144). Although a hemorrhagic or discolored aspirant is the rule for cysts containing tumors, at least 6 patients have been reported in the literature in whom clear cyst fluid had been aspi-

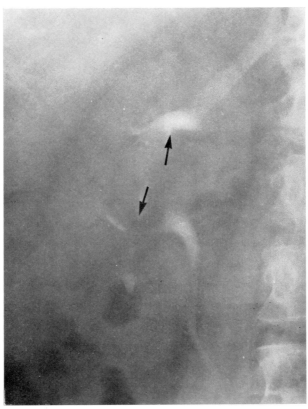

Figure 46a, b, c, d, e. Successive intravenous pyelograms demonstrate progressive enlargement of a space-occupying lesion in the right kidney over several years. There is evidence of displacement and splaying of infundibula and calyces on the first intravenous pyelogram. On the later pyelogram, one questions destruction of the midcalyceal group. In general, however, the characteristics were suggestive of a progressively enlarging renal cyst.

A flush aortogram demonstrates a spherical, relatively avascular lesion in the midportion of the right kidney corresponding to the defect suggested on the intravenous pyelogram. A questionable stain along the superior circumference of the lesion as well as some puddling of contrast medium raises the question of a cystic tumor (arrows).

A selective renal arteriogram after pre-injection of adrenalin hydrochloride demonstrates clusters of abnormal vessels arranged in a spherical pattern. This appearance suggested that the vessels might be lining the inner circumference of a globe-like structure. Note the "spur" at the interface of normal parenchyma and mass (arrow) presumed diagnostic for a renal cyst. Cyst puncture and aspiration further affirmed the presence of a tumor arising from the lining of a cyst wall and demonstrated extravasation between layers of tumor. (Pathologically: Tumor of cyst lining)

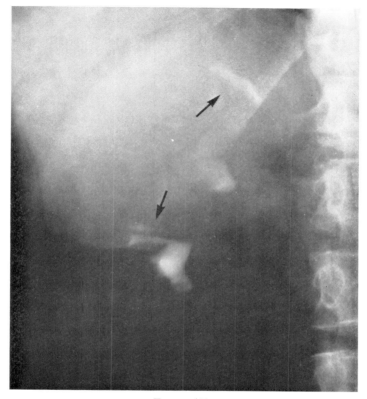

FIGURE 46b.

rated from a cyst containing a proven tumor (17, 18, 42, 81, 148, 231). Conversely, hemorrhagic or discolored fluid has been aspirated from proven benign simple serous cysts (144).

In our experience, histochemical and histopathological assessment of the aspirated fluid proved to be highly reliable (Table XIII). In 3 patients, the tumor protruded directly into the lumen of the cyst. The aspirant was highly hemorrhagic, the fat content of the aspirant high, and the Papanicolaou smear positive in all 3 patients. Pathological examination of the removed specimen showed the cyst to be lined by normal serous epithelium with the exception of a friable tumor mass protruding into the cyst in one patient from the base of the cyst and, in two other patients, from the

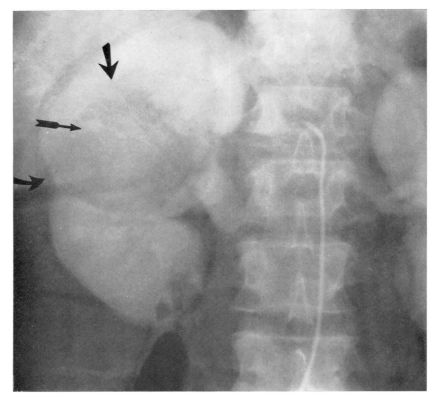

FIGURE 46c.

dependent margin of the cyst. The tumor that arose from the base of the cyst was readily demonstrable on a selective renal arteriogram after injection of adrenalin hydrochloride. The two tumors arising from the dependent circumference of the cyst wall were quite avascular and failed to show any tumor stain or demonstrate any abnormal vessels. Scintiscanograms, nephrotomograms, intravenous pyelograms, and retrograde pyelograms suggested the presence of a space-occupying lesion but in no way indicated the presence of a tumor. The double contrast studies demonstrated filling defects in all three of these cysts (Fig. 50a, b, c). The diagnosis was confirmed on basis of the histochemical and histopatho-

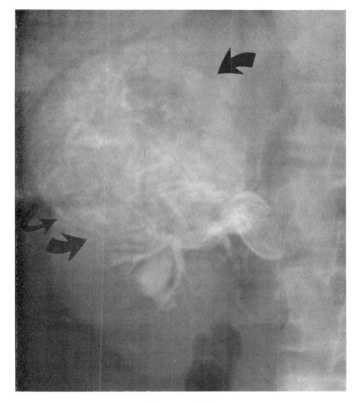

FIGURE 46d.

logical findings of the aspirant and the roentgenographic demonstration of a mass lesion projecting into the opacified cyst (Table XIV) (164).

In two of our patients, the tumor appeared to arise within the layers of the cyst wall (Table XIV). Microscopic examination of both specimen revealed infiltration of the inner lining of the cyst by several layers of clear cells typical of carcinoma. The fluid aspirated by percutaneous cyst puncture was cloudy in both patients. Papanicolaou smear was unequivocally positive for tumor in one patient, in the other a questionable grade was assigned. The fat content was high in the patient with the positive Papanico-

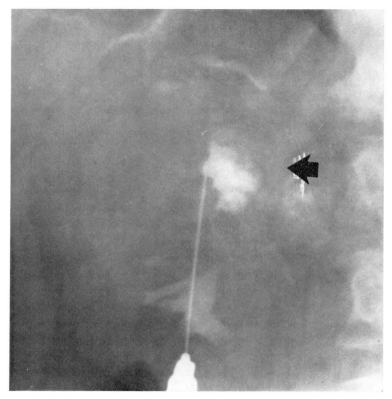

FIGURE 46e.

laou smear but was low in the patient with the questionable Papanicolaou grade. Fortunately, however, the unquestionable diagnosis of neoplasm could be made on basis of the selective renal arteriogram. Clusters of abnormal vessels appeared to surround the periphery of a spherical mass lesion (Fig. 46a, b, c, d, e). In one of the patients, the characteristic findings of veins draining a tumor were demonstrated on a venogram of the plexus enveloping the cystic lesion (Fig. 49a, b).

One of these patients is of particular interest since he had been followed periodically for five years with intravenous urograms for the presumed diagnosis of renal cyst. Over this period, the intravenous urogram demonstrated doubling of the cross diameter of

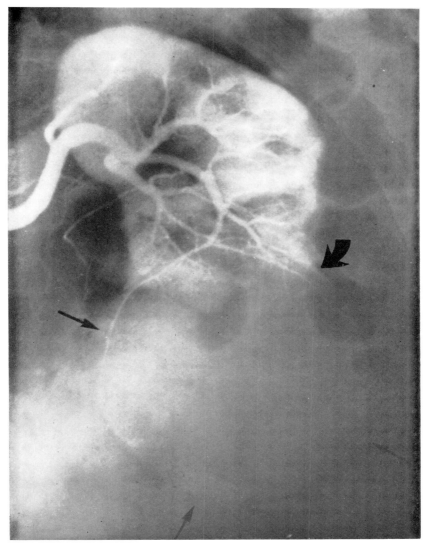

FIGURE 47a, b. A selective renal arteriogram demonstrates an avascular lesion in the lower pole of the left kidney. Note the characteristic splaying and displacement of branch vessels and the demonstration of a well demarcated interphase suggesting a benign cyst. A cyst puncture disclosed murky and grossly bloody aspirant. The injection of contrast material resulted in a typical intraparenchymal distribution pattern of a tumor. The retrograde pyelogram performed for identification of the kidney demonstrated globular distortion of the inferior calyceal group. A tumor was found in the base of a cystic structure at exploration. (Courtesy, Lang — Journal of Urology.)

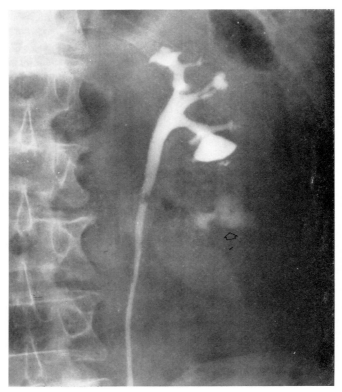

FIGURE 47b.

this space-occupying lesion in the mid section of the kidney. However, at no time was there any other pyelographic evidence suggesting a neoplastic entity. A translumbar aortogram had been performed when the patient was first seen and an avascular lesion quite typical of a renal cyst had been demonstrated. The flush arteriogram and nephrotomogram at the time of final diagnosis confirmed once more an avascular lesion with arteriographic and nephrotomographic characteristics of a benign cyst. A thin wall was readily identified on the nephrotomogram and the interface between the avascular lesion and the staining renal parenchyma was sharply delineated. A typical parenchymal "spur" marked the cortical margin of the presumed benign cyst. A selective renal arteriogram, pre-empted by injection of adrenalin hydrochloride in one patient and glucagon in the other patient, however, demonstrated abnormal vessels lining the mass in a globe-like fashion (Fig. 46a, b, c, d, e). Although the tumor did not protrude into the lumen of the cyst, a peculiar coating of the inner surface of the cyst wall was demonstrated on double contrast cyst studies. This peculiar "coating effect" suggested an abnormal surface. Examination of the specimen confirmed infiltration of the

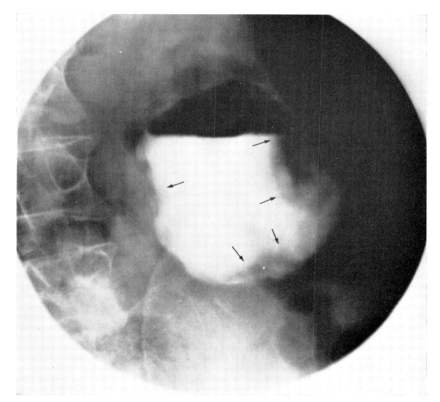

FIGURE 48a, b, c. A double contrast cyst study demonstrates multiple filing defects projecting into the lumen of the cyst. Histochemical and histopathological examination of the bloody aspirant confirmed the presence of a tumor. The surgical specimen demonstrated multiple friable tumor nodules protruding into the lumen of the cyst but apparently originating from the cyst wall. (Courtesy, Lang — Journal of Urology.)

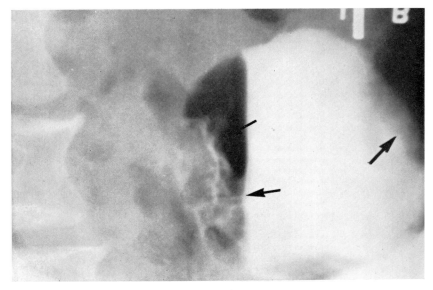

FIGURE 48b.

inner surface by layers of carcinoma with fibrin deposit coating the areas of tumor penetration. It is postulated that the "coating effect" by Hypaque was facilitated by these fibrin deposits (164).

The origin of neoplasms between the septas of a multilocular cyst or in a polycystic kidney has been established in the recent literature (42, 82, 134, 148, 171). Khorsand reported a neoplasm in the common base of two cystic cavities, both of which contained yellowish clear fluid (148). Brannan and Howard emphasized the occurrence of renal neoplasms in polycystic kidneys (42, 134).

The diagnosis of such a lesion in a multilocular cyst is particularly difficult. As a rule, such tumors are so small that demonstration by selective renal arteriograms may be arduous. The demonstration of compartments of multilocular cysts by double contrast cyst study in itself may be quite difficult and may necessitate multiple punctures to obtain filling of the entire mass as delineated on nephrotomograms or renal arteriograms (Table VI) (Fig. 45a, b). The demonstration of a small tumor arising

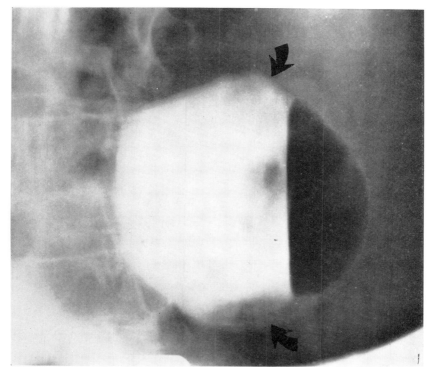

FIGURE 48c.

between the septas of such multilocular cysts is extremely difficult. For this reason, one has to rely primarily on the histochemical and histopathological examination of the aspirated fluid (148).

Selective renal angiography, particularly in conjunction with certain pharmacologic agents, can be relied upon for the diagnosis of renal cell carcinoma in polycystic disease. Similar to the experience related by Howard, we were able to diagnose a renal cell carcinoma in the lower pole of a polycystic kidney (134, 164). A selective arteriogram of the lower polar artery demonstrated a sustained arteriographic stain, however, corkscrew vessels or puddling of dye was not seen. Exploration revealed a relatively small renal cell carcinoma arising from the renal parenchyma between several large and small cysts. The tumor protruded into the lumen of at least one large and two small cysts. It was of interest to note that the gross specimen showed bluish discoloration of all cysts

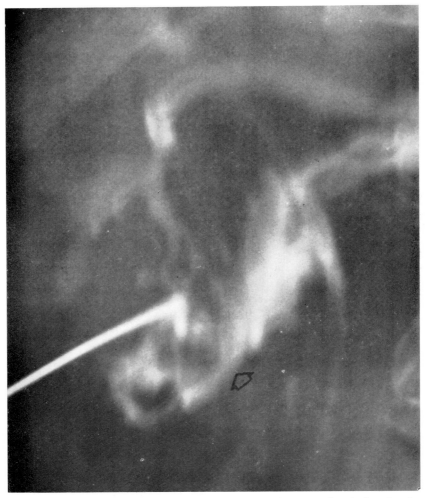

FIGURE 49a, b. A percutaneous puncture of a cystic appearing lesion in the lower pole of the right kidney was attempted. After placement of the needle, venous blood was readily aspirated and a selective venogram was carried out. The demonstrated venous channels are characteristic of the veins in the rim of a hypernephroma. Note the massive size of the circumferential veins and the dual drainage pattern via two major branch veins. (Courtesy, Lang — Journal of Urology.)

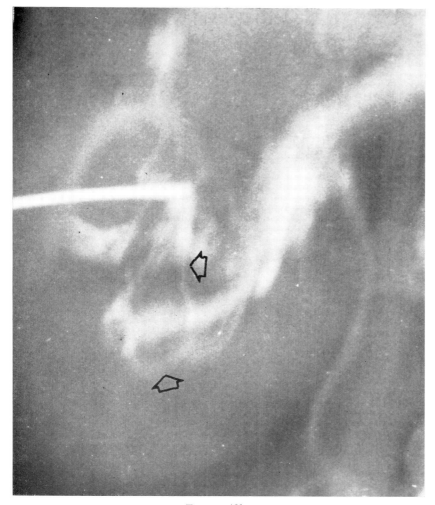

FIGURE 49b.

which were involved by tumor. Aspiration from these cysts revealed a grossly bloody fluid. The fluid in the other cysts in the
upper pole and mid portion of the removed kidney was slightly
yellowish but clear.

The presence of filling defects in the kidney pelvis, infundibula and calyces in patients with known multilocular cysts should

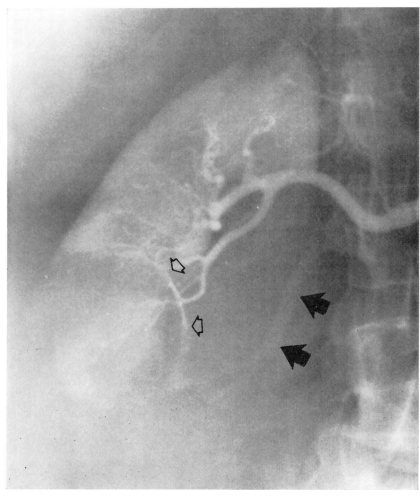

FIGURE 50a, b, c. A selective right renal arteriogram demonstrates splaying of interlobar vessels around what appears to be a spherical mass lesion in the lower one-half of the right kidney. Note the perpendicular entry of some vessels into this mass lesion and an extremely early opacification of draining veins raising the question of a renal neoplasm with arteriovenous shunts. A nephrographic phase roentgenogram demonstrates an area of increased stain of the interface between this cystic mass lesion and the adjacent renal parenchyma. The lower pole and medial sector of the kidney were supplied by separate vessels. Note evidence of puddling of contrast medium in the center of this cystic lesion. A cyst puncture and aspiration revealed the presence of grossly bloody and murky aspirant. Injection with contrast medium demonstrated a relatively smooth central cystic cavity and extravasation of contrast medium into the surrounding necrotic hypernephroma.

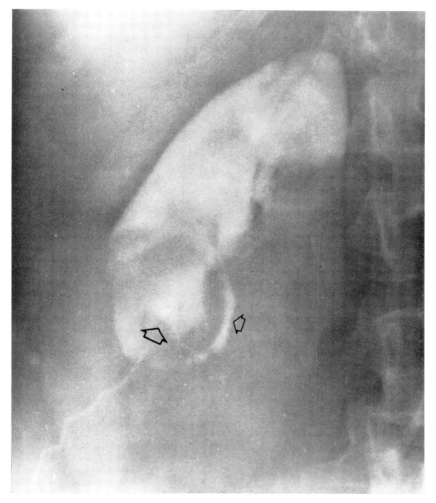

FIGURE 50b.

be evaluated with great care. Smooth curvilinear filling defects
readily demonstrable or intravenous urography and retrograde
pyelography usually reflect intrapelvic herniation of daughter
cysts rather than a neoplastic mass (268) .

The fourth type of coexistence of renal carcinoma and
renal cyst is based on the geographic and etiologic relationship of

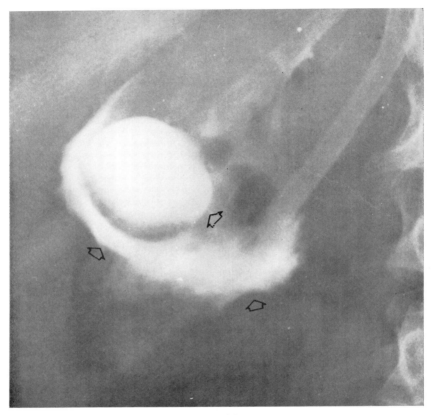

FIGURE 50c.

these two lesions. Following the theory advanced by Hepler that obstruction of arterial supply and tubules may cause cysts, Gibson postulated that a tumor may likewise cause such a cyst (110, 130). Accepting this theoretical axiom, the tumor would have to be located in the base of the cyst. While this relationship has not been observed very frequently, there are at least ten reported cases including one of our own that would meet these criteria (18, 42, 76, 77, 81, 144, 148, 164, 280).

On basis of the composite experience reported in the literature, coexistence of renal carcinoma and cysts can be successfully diagnosed by today's diagnostic techniques. The flat plate of the

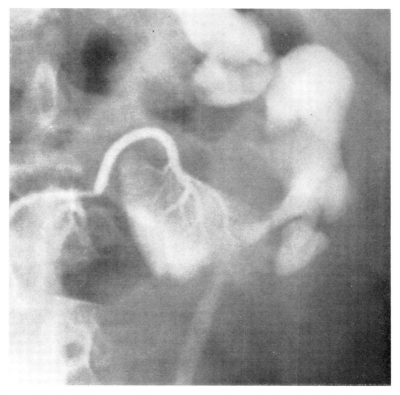

FIGURE 51a, b. The composite superimposition of selective injections of several renal arteries supplying the left kidney demonstrates an avascular mass in central position. Exploration confirmed the presence of a central cyst in a malrotated kidney.

abdomen, the intravenous urogram, the nephrotomogram, and the scintiscanogram are unable to identify such a combination of lesions other than the accidental occurrence of a renal carcinoma and renal cyst in the same kidney but widely separated. However, carefully performed selective renal arteriograms augmented by injection of adrenalin hydrochloride or glucagon should be capable of demonstrating abnormal vessels in all cystic and necrotic hypernephromas and in most carcinomas arising from the lining of a cyst or protruding into the lumen of a cyst. A definitive diagnosis

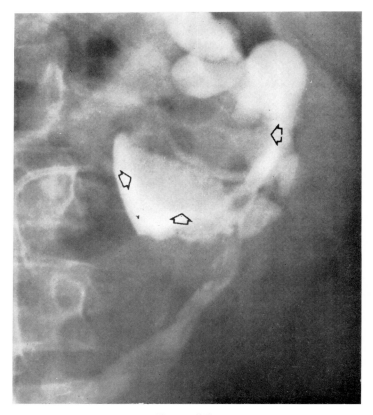

FIGURE 51b.

of coexistence of cysts and tumor can be established on basis of a demonstrable filling defect on double contrast cyst studies and on basis of the tell-tale results of histochemical and histopathological examination of the aspirant. It is, however, admitted that our present day criteria will not permit differentiation of malignant versus benign tumor associated with a cyst. Cystic hamartoma and adenomyoma will present an indistinguishable pattern on arteriogram and on double contrast study and the cyst aspirant may frequently show a hemorrhagic cyst fluid with high fat content (188).

It is felt that composite assessment by roentgenographic, histochemical and histopathological techniques permits diagnosis of renal cysts, neoplasms, or any combination with an adequate degree of accuracy to forego surgical exploration once held obligatory in the management of these lesions.

CHAPTER V

TECHNIQUE

NEPHROTOMOGRAPHY, RENAL ANGIOGRAPHY, retroperitoneal gas studies, and cyst puncture, aspiration and double contrast demonstration of renal cysts are mutually complementary examinations designed to establish a definitive diagnosis of the type of renal mass lesion. The choice of sequence and technique of these studies is of critical importance for speedy completion of each segment of this battery of tests. The procedures must be performed with a minimum of trauma to eliminate recovery periods resulting from undue trauma of each procedure. Certain procedures mutually enhancing their respective diagnostic value should be performed simultaneously. Concomitant retroperitoneal gas study and selective renal angiography has been advocated for optimal assessment of tumor penetration through the capsule of the kidney and to improve roentgenographic small vessel detail.

RETROPERITONEAL GAS STUDY

After proper cleaning of the perineum, 2 percent Xylocaine is instilled as local anesthetic. An 18-gauge $3\frac{1}{2}$ inch long needle is introduced into the presacral space. Advancement of the needle and placement of the tip above the roof of the levator anus is monitored by a finger introduced into the rectum. One thousand to fifteen hundred cc of carbon dioxide or four thousand to six thousand cc of nitrous oxide are then insufflated. For optimal dissection along the psoas muscle, the patient is rotated from a prone position into the 45° oblique decubitus position, elevating the table to a 30° to 45° semiupright position. The progress of dissection can be monitored fluoroscopically. Dissection is continued until a clear margin of the suprarenal gland or the tumor

148

mass of the kidney is discernible fluoroscopically. The relatively slow reabsorption of nitrous oxide from the retroperitoneal space permits in addition unhurried renal arteriography. The introduction of gas into the retroperitoneal space effects a desirable change of the physical characteristics facilitating roentgenographic demonstration of small vessels. Cannibalism of extra-renal systems and the development of collateral vessels between the capsular arteries, the lumbar arteries, the subcostal and phrenic arteries may be best appreciated on such combined studies (159, 163).

ARTERIOGRAPHY OF RENAL MASS LESIONS

After prepping and draping an appropriate area of the groin, 2 percent Xylocaine® solution is instilled for local anesthesia. A small incision is made at the intended point of skin puncture and the subcutaneous tissues are spread with a hemostat to facilitate subsequent passage of the catheter. A meticulous percutaneous puncture of the femoral artery is then carried out and a wire inserted through the outer sheath of this thin-walled trocar needle. The catheter, with the tip molded to a J-shaped configuration, is threaded over the wire. Catheter and wire, the highly flexible tip of the wire leading by approximately 15 cm are advanced into the abdominal aorta under fluoroscopic control. After removal of the guidewire, the catheter tip resumes its J-shaped configuration facilitating engagement of the renal arteries.

Selective engagement of both renal arteries is carried out and the position confirmed fluoroscopically by monitoring of injections of 2 to 3 cc of 50 percent sodium diatrizoate (156).

Hand injections of 8 to 15 cc of 50 percent sodium diatrizoate suffice for excellent opacification of the renal artery. The injection should be prolonged over a period of 2 to 3 seconds and the events recorded on serial roentgenograms covering a total period of 12 to 15 seconds. The initial arterial phase is best recorded at a rate of no less than 4 exposures per second; the late phase is adequately documented at a rate of 1 exposure per second. AP and lateral projections and, in some instances, posterior oblique projections are favored for optimal demonstration.

Patients suspected of renal tumor or tumors associated with

renal cysts are injected a second time using 15 cc of sodium diatrizoate preceded by a selective intra-arterial injection of 10 cc of
adrenalin hydrochloride solution containing 1µg per ml (3, 142).
The lack of response to adrenalin by tumor vessels contrasted to
the marked constriction of normal vessels results in better appreci-
ation of sparse tumor vessels. Many necrotic tumors or tumors in
renal cysts may show abnormal tumor vessels only after the com-
petition with the normal vascularity has been eliminated by con-
stricting these vessels with adrenalin hydrochloride. Because of
the marked retardation of flow resulting from increased peripheral arterial resistance, the speed of injection has to be slowed and
the roentgenographic documentation prolonged to cover a period
of no less than 20 seconds. The rate of exposure of 1 per second
for the first 10 seconds and 1 per every 2 seconds for the last 10-
second period suffices for adequate recording of the events.

If one suspects invasion of the renal vein by tumor, another
injection with 20 to 30 cc of contrast medium, preferably of higher iodine concentration such as sodium iothalamate 80 percent,
sodium meglumine, or meglumine iothalamate is suggested. Even
though such a large bolus of contrast medium may cause a renal
shutdown, this risk appears justified since the presence of a tumor
has already been established, surgical removal decided and, particularly, since the selection of appropriate techniques for surgical
extirpation depends on the preoperative determination of the
presence or absence of renal vein or inferior vena cava invasion by
tumor. The injection of a large bolus of contrast medium of high
iodine concentration produces adequate opacification of the renal
vein to permit assessment for the presence or absence of tumor
implants. The roentgenographic documentation should emphasize the venous phase and a recording rate of 1 per second for the
first 5 seconds and 2 per second for the subsequent 8 seconds is
favored (165).

After completion of the selective studies of the renal arteries, a
flush injection of the aorta is mandatory for demonstration of
cannibalism of the vascular supply of adjacent organs by a tumor
that may have extended into adjacent tissues.

For this purpose, the catheter is placed approximately $2\frac{1}{2}$

inches above the origin of the renal arteries and 30 to 50 cc of contrast medium, preferably of high iodine concentration are injected utilizing a pressure syringe. The injection pressure is adjusted to deliver the entire bolus in 1.8 to 2.5 seconds. To avoid substitution of catheters during the procedure, the J-shaped catheter is equipped with four side-holes to prevent undesirable "whipping" during the pressure injection. Roentgenographic documentation is best obtained on serial roentgenograms covering a period of some 15 seconds. An exposure rate of 2 per second for the first 4 seconds and 1 per second for the remainder guarantees adequate coverage.

Selective injection of lumbar, adrenal, subcostal, phrenic, spermatic, and hepatic arteries should be carried out if the flush injection suggests vascular supply of tumor elements by any of these vessel groups (38, 148, 140, 141, 165). Engagement of these vessels can be accomplished without change of catheter. By extending the flexible J-shaped guidewire beyond the tip of the catheter for varying lengths, an indefinite number of different configurations can be created, facilitating engagement of various vessels. Injections of 5 to 7 cc of 50 percent sodium diatrizoate afford excellent visualization of the lumbar, intercostal, subcostal, phrenic, and adrenal arteries. If a tumor derives predominant supply from one of these vessels, a larger amount of contrast medium is necessary to obtain optimal opacification. Fifteen to thirty cc of contrast medium afford optimal opacification of the selectively engaged hepatic artery. The events are best recorded at a rate of 4 roentgenograms per second for the first 3 seconds and 2 per second for the remaining 9 seconds.

Stringent adherence to the proposed table of examination permits the physician to stay within limits of contrast medium tolerance. Maximal amounts of contrast medium used to complete the gamut of selective flush injections should not exceed 100 cc in an adult patient.

Manual compression of the puncture site after removal of the arterial catheter and application of a proper pressure dressing minimize postoperative complications. The intra-arterial instillation of 20 to 50 mg of Heparin immediately prior to removal of the catheter has decreased the occurrence of venous complications such as thrombophlebitis. Meticulous postoperative follow-up care is mandatory to recognize postoperative complications at an early time and prevent development of serious complications by prompt institution of appropriate therapy (156, 160) .

CYST PUNCTURE, ASPIRATION AND DOUBLE CONTRAST STUDIES OF CYSTS

The mass known from previous excretory or retrograde urograms is identified fluoroscopically some 10 to 15 minutes after intravenous injection of a urographic contrast medium. A radiopaque marker is placed on the prone patient. An appropriate area is then cleaned, prepped and draped and a generous wheal of local anesthetic is made in the skin at the marked point. Infiltration with anesthetic medium is extended to one to two inches below the skin. A 20-gauge thin-walled short beveled needle is inserted via translumbar approach and under fluoroscopic control advanced into the mass. The puncture is carried out in one brisk motion during which time the patient is admonished to desist from breathing. Occasionally, penetration of fascia and even cyst wall may be identifiable to touch transmitted by the needle. After removal of the stylus, a malleable plastic tubing is attached to allow free excursion of the needle following respiratory motion of the kidney during the process of fluid aspiration and instillation of contrast medium and air. The fluid usually evacuates slowly through the lumen of the needle. If no fluid can be aspirated, the needle should be left in position and another set of roentgenograms in AP and lateral projection should be obtained to determine the exact position of the tip of the needle in reference to the renal mass. If the fluoroscope is equipped with a C-arm, the position of the needle in relation to the mass can be ascertained by merely rotating the fluoroscopic device 90°. Failure of aspiration of fluid from a mass with known correct position of the needle tip may be considered evidence for the diagnosis of a neoplasm. Contrast medium may be injected to demonstrate the interstitial distribution of the radiopaque medium in a solid tumor mass (Fig. 46c, 50c) . Frequently, a few drops of fluid can be aspirated from such a mass and subsequently utilized for cytologic examination. However, even if this is not possible, a needle biopsy may be obtained by applying strong suction to the syringe while removing the needle (216). Aspiration of blood or discolored fluid suggests puncture of a necrotic tumor mass, a cyst containing tumor, a cyst with preceding hemorrhage, or possibly merely a traumatic tap. Even though it has been advocated in the past to terminate the procedure if a bloody or discolored aspirant was encountered, we now proceed with instillation of contrast medium and gas to obtain a double contrast study of the cavity (160, 216, 222, 286).

No attempt is made to completely evacuate the cyst, however, an adequate sample of cyst fluid is obtained to permit histochemical and histopathological study. The amount aspirated is replaced by contrast medium and air or gas. Equal volume replacement of the aspirant by air and contrast medium is important to reconstruct the pre-existing anatomical conditions for appropriate correlation with preceding intravenous urograms, nephrotomograms, or arteriographic studies.

Atraumatic withdrawal of the needle is accomplished by removal in one brisk motion, again admonishing the patient to desist from breathing during this procedure. The danger of tearing renal parenchymal substance or capsule is thus minimized. After removal of the needle, roentgenograms are obtained in prone, supine, lateral decubitus, upright, 45° Trendelenburg, and oblique positions. Each wall segment of the cyst or compound cyst is thus demonstrated on double contrast air cystograms. Protrusion of a mass into the lumen of the cyst should be demonstrable in at least one of these standard projections. Tomography of the opacified cyst may be added to permit demonstration of the cyst wall at various levels in great detail (144). The roentgenograms obtained after double contrast cyst study should be superimposed upon an identical AP and lateral projection of a preceding arteriogram or nephrotomogram. The opacified cyst should correspond to the negative defect demonstrated on arteriogram or nephrotomogram. If this correlation test identifies other unexplained areas of decreased stain on the nephrographic phase roentgenogram, further attempts to puncture these mass lesions should be undertaken. In several instances, this correlation led to discovery of small satellite cysts and, in at least one patient in our series disclosed an unrelated tumor (163, 164, 169).

An attempt to completely empty the cyst by aspiration was advocated by Phillips but is no longer widely practiced (222). The author emphasized that the pyelocalyceal pattern should return to normal after collapse of the simple cyst and advocated this phenomenon as a reliable diagnostic criterion for excluding the presence of other mass lesions. Therapeutic evacuation of renal cysts or instillation of sclerosing media is likewise advocated only sparingly (280).

76. Edholm, P.: Roentgen diagnosis of expansive processes in the kidneys. Nord. Med. 66:1497-1500, 1961. (Sw)

77. Edholm, P., Fernstrom, I., Lindblom, K., and Seldinger, S.I.: Roentgen television in practice with special regard to puncture examination. Acta Radiol (suppl) 216, 1962.

78. Edsman, G.: Angionephrography in malignant renal tumors. Urol Int 6: 117-125, 1958.

79. Eggers, H., and Strohmann, G.: Uber dysplastische cystoide Nierenblastome. Z Urol 57:877-885, 1964.

80. Eisenman, J.I., Finck, R.R., and Girdany, B.R.: Collateral vein sign: angiographic demonstration of renal vein invasion in renal carcinoma. Radiology 92:1256-1261, 1969.

81. Emanuel, M.: Small renal cell carcinoma presenting as solitary cyst. J Maine Med Assoc 44:192-195, 1953.

82. Emmett, J.L., Levine, S.R., and Woolner, L.B.: Co-existence of renal cyst and tumour: incidence in 1,007 cases. Brit J Urol 35:403-410, 1963.

83. Emmett, J.L.: Clinical urography. Vol 2, 2nd ed, W. B. Saunders Co, Philadelphia, 1964.

84. Ettinger, A., and Elkin, M.: Value of plain film in renal mass lesions (Tumors and cysts). Radiology 62:372-382, 1954.

85. Ettinger, A., and Robbins, A.H.: Detection of small renal tumors. Am J Roentgenol 104:335-342, 1968.

86. Ettinger, A., Kahn, P.C., and Wise, H.M., Jr.: Importance of selective renal angiography in diagnosis of polycystic disease. J Urol 102: 156-161, 1969.

87. Evans, J.A., Dubilier, W., Jr., and Monteith, J.C.: Nephrotomography: A preliminary report. Amer J Roentgenol 71:213-223, 1954.

88. Evans, J.A., Monteith, J.C., and Dubilier, W., Jr.: Nephrotomography. Radiology 64:655-663, 1955.

89. Evans, J.A.: Nephrotomography in the investigation of renal masses. Radiology 69:684-689, 1957.

90. Evans, J.A., Halpern, M., and Finley, N.: Diagnosis of kidney cancer: An analysis of 100 consecutive cases. JAMA 175:201-203, 1961.

91. Evans, J.: The accuracy of diagnostic radiology. JAMA 204:131-134, 1968.

92. Everson, T.C.: Spontaneous regression of cancer. Ann N Y Acad Sci 114:721-735, 1964.

93. Ferreira-Berrutti, P., and Porta, G.: Lipangioleiomioma del rinon (associado con esclerosis tuberosa). An Fac Med Montev 49:349-355, 1964.

94. Fetter, T.R., Yunen, J.R., and Bogaev, J.H.: Parapelvic renal cyst: report of three additional cases. J Urol 88:599-603, 1962.

95. Fetter, T.R., and Snyder, A.I.: Survival study in renal cell carcinoma. Surg Gynec and Obst 117:7-9, 1963.

96. Fiedler, H.T.: Hypernephroma presenting clinically and roentgenologically as a solitary cyst. Z Urol 56:207, 1963. (Ger.)

· 97. Fine, M.G.: Intrapelvic presentation of renal cysts: report of two cases and discussion of the literature. J Urol 91:325-329, 1964.

98. Fishbone, G., and Davidson, A.J.: Leiomyoma of the renal capsule. Radiology 92:1006-1007, 1969.

99. Flocks, R.H., and Kadesky, H.C.: Malignant neoplasms of the kidney: An analysis of 353 patients followed for 3 years or more. Trans Amer Assoc Genito-Urin Surg 49:105-110, 1957.

100. Folin, J.: Roentgenography without contrast medium and urography in the diagnosis of kidney tumors. Radiologe (Berlin) 1:166-170, 1961. (Ger)

101. Freed, S.Z., Caplan, L.H., and Bosniak, M.A.: The role of renal arteriography in the management of renal carcinoma. Surg Gynec Obst 123:1303-1308, 1966.

102. Frimann-Dahl, J.: Radiology in renal cysts particularly on left side. Brit J Radiol. 37:146-153, 1964.

103. Frimann-Dahl, J.: Angiography in renal tumors and cysts: Renal angiography. Kincaid, O.W., and Davis, G.D. Year Book Publishers, Chicago, 1966.

104. Gamba, A., and Cillo, L.: Le cisti dermoidi del rene. Chir. Ital 16:68-87, 1964.

105. Gaentzen, F.J.: Parapelvic renal cysts. Ztschr Urol 53:371-376, 1960.

106. George, R., and Franchisk, F.: A case of cystic hemangioma of the cerebellum (lindau tumor) with the presence of simultaneous metastasis of hypernephroma in the cerebellum. Zr Nevropat Psikhiat Korsakov 61:1644-1649, 1961. (Rus)

107. Gerasimenko, P.P.: Arterial hypertension in patients with renal tumors and cysts. Ter Arkh 37:65-71, 1965. (Rus)

108. Gernert, J.E., Stein, J., and Bischoff, A.J.: Solitary renal cysts: experience with 100 cases. J Urol 100:251-253, 1968.

109. Giampalmo, A., and Piazza, M.: Gli-angiomi del rene. Minerva Nefrol 10:133-134, 1963.

110. Gibson, T.E.: Interrelationship of renal cysts and tumors. Report of three cases. J Urol 71:241-252, 1954.

111. Gordon, A.: Renal glomerular adenomatosis. J Path Bact 83:555-557, 1962.

112. Goria, A.: Solitary cysts of the kidney. Arch Sci Med (Tor) 108:723-754, 1959. (It)

113. Gosfay, S.: Xanthomatos degenerierendes Neurofibrom im Nierenstiel. Acta Chir Acad Sci Hung 5:83-86, 1964.

114. Grabstald, H.: The extent of nephrectomy for renal cell cancer. JAMA 204:227-229, 1968.

115. Greene, L.F., Witten, D.M., and Emmett, J.L.: Nephrotomography in urologic diagnosis. J Urol 91:184-189, 1964.

116. Gregg, D.: Renal and suprarenal tumours in adults. Brit J Radiol 37: 128-141, 1964.

117. Griscom, N.T.: The roentgenology of neonatal abdominal masses. Amer J Roentgenol 93:447-463, 1965.

·118. Grossman, H., Winchester, P.H., and Chisari, F. V.: Roentgenographic classification of renal cystic disease. Am J Roentgenol 104:319-331, 1968.

119. Guillemin, P.: Cysts of the renal hilus. J Urol Nephrol (Paris) 68:715-720, 1962. (Fr)

120. Hagen, A.: Renal angioma. Four cases of angioma of the renal pelvis. Acta Chir Scand 126: 657-667, 1963.

121. Hajdu, S.I., and Thomas, A.G.: Renal cell carcinoma at autopsy. J Urol 97:978-982, 1967.

122. Hajos, E.: On roentgen differential diagnosis of kidney tumors. Radiol Diagn (Berlin) 2:289-301, 1961. (Ger)

123. Harvard, B.M., and Evans, J.S.: Simultaneous bilateral transitional cell carcinoma of the renal pelvis. J Urol 91:14-19, 1964.

124. Hayashi, Y., Shimizu, S., and Takizawa, H.: Case report: pyelogenic cyst secondary to localized obliterating pyelonephritis. Jap J Urol 54: 520-526, 1963. (Jap)

125. Hayward, W.G.: Hypernephroma in a polycystic kidney. J Urol 56:190-192, 1946.

126. Hemley, S.D., Arida, E.J., and Finby, N.: Nephrotomography: Its practical advantages. J Urol 90:510-513, 1963.

127. Hengst, W.: Tumordiagnostik mit radioaktiven Quecksilberverbindungen. Med Klin 60:1929-1932, 1965.

128. Henken, E.M.: "Milk of Calcium" in a renal cyst: report of a case. Radiology 84:276-278, 1965.

129. Henthorne, J.G.: Peripelvic lymphatic cysts of kidney: Review of literature on perinephric cysts. Am J Clin Path. 8:28-38, 1950.

130. Hepler, A.B.: Solitary cysts of the kidney: a report of seven cases and observations on the pathogenesis of these cysts. Surg Gynec Obst 50:668-687, 1930.

131. Hickey, B.B., Evans, C.J., Sharp, M.E., and Ashley, D.J.: Renal and pulmonary tuberous sclerosis: the relationship of the renal lesion to haemangiopericytoma. Brit J Surg 49:396-400, 1962.

132. Hierholzer, G., and Rehn, J.: Perirenale Riesencyste nach stumpfem Nierentrauma. Beitrag zum Problem der stumpfel Nierenverletzugen. Unfallheilk 67:272-278, 1964.

133. Hoffman, R., and Riley, J.: The diagnostic approach to the parenchymal renal mass. Am J Roentgenol 100:698-708, 1967.

134. Howard, R.M., and Young, J.D., Jr.: Two malignant tumors in polycystic kidney. J Urol 102:162-164, 1969.

135. Howell, R.D.: Milk of calcium renal stone. J Urol 82:197-199, 1959.

136. Iozzi, L., Blocklyn, M., and Rosenberg, F.: Renal milk of calcium stone. J Urol 93:556-558, 1965.
137. Jalundhwala, J.M., and Shah, R.C.: Traumatic perinephric cyst. Brit J Urol 35:133-136, 1963.
138. Jantet, G.H., Foot, E.C., and Kenyon, J.R.: Rupture of an intrarenal arteriovenous fistula secondary to carcinoma: a case report. Brit J Surg 49:404-406, 1962.
139. Johnson, W.F.: Carcinoma in a polycystic kidney. J Urol 69:10-12, 1953.
140. Kahn, P.C.: Selective angiography of the inferior phrenic arteries. Radiology 88:1-8, 1967.
141. Kahn, P.C., Wise, H.M., and Robbins, A.H.: Complete angiographic evaluation of renal cancer. JAMA 204:753-757, 1968.
142. Kahn, P.C., and Wise, H.M.: The use of epinephrine in selective angiography of renal masses. J Urol 99:133-138, 1968.
143. Kahn, P.C.: Selective venography in renal parenchymal disease. Radiology 92:345-349, 1969.
144. Kaiser, T.F., Hodsen, G.M., Seibel, R.E., Albee, R.D., Farrow, F.C., and McMahon, J.J.: Evaluation of asymptomatic renal masses by selective renal angiography and percutaneous needle puncture: a preliminary report. J Urol 98:436-443, 1967.
145. Kaufman, J.J.: Reasons for nephrectomy. JAMA 207:145-146, 1968.
146. Kaufman, J.J., and Mims, M.D.: Tumors of the kidney in "Current problems in surgery." Chicago Year Book Med Publ, pp. 1-44, Feb 1966.
147. Khilnani, M.T., and Wolf, B.S.: Hamartolipoma of the kidney: clinical and roentgen features. Amer J Roentgenol 86:830-841, 1961.
148. Khorsand, D.: Carcinoma within solitary renal cysts. J Urol 93: 440-444, 1965.
149. King, M.C., Friedenberg, R.M., and Tena, L.B.: Normal renal parenchyma simulating tumor. Radiology 91:217-222, 1968.
150. Klapproth, H.J., Poutasse, E.F., and Hazard, J.B.: Renal angiomyelipomas — mixed mesenchymal hamartomas. AMA Arch Path 67: 400-411, 1959.
151. Klosterhalfen, H.: Zur Differentialdiagnose Nierentumoren-Nierencyste mit Hilfe der Renocystographie. Z Urol 56:419-422, 1963.
152. Kotlarek-Haus, S., Gabrys, K., and Kiszkiel, K.: Appearance of a calcified cyst and a carcinoma in the same kidney. Pol Tyg Lek 21:142-144, 1966. (Pol)
153. Krentzmann, H.A.: Hypertension associated with solitary renal cyst: report of 2 cases. J Urol 57:467-472, 1947.
154. Lalli, A.F.: The roentgen diagnosis of renal cyst and tumor. J Canad Assoc Radiol 17:41-43, 1966.
155. Lamarina, A.: Il Leiomioma maligno o Leiomisarcoma del rene. (Conoscenze attulai e contributo casistico). Osped Maggiore 59:595-611, 1964.

156. Lang, E.K.: A survey of the complications of percutaneous retrograde arteriography. Radiology 81:257-263, 1963.

157. Lang, E.K.: Direct needle puncture in the diagnosis of renal mass lesions in infants. J Ind St Med Assoc 58:143-144, 1965.

158. Lang, E.K.: The differential diagnosis of renal cysts and tumor. Cyst puncture, aspiration, and analysis of cyst content for fat as diagnostic criteria for renal cysts. Radiology 87:457-461, 1966.

159. Lang, E.K.: Diagnosis of suprarenal mass lesions by retroperitoneal gas studies and arteriography. Radiology 87:35-45, 1966.

160. Lang, E.K.: Prevention and treatment of complications following arteriography. Radiology 88:950-956, 1967.

161. Lang, E.K.: Aneurysms and arteriovenous fistulae in a hypernephroma. J Ind St Med Assoc 62:276-277, 1969.

162. Lang, E.K.: Superselective arterial catheterization of tumors of the genitourinary tract: a modality used for perfusion with chemotherapeutic agents and infarction with radioactive pellets. J Urol (in print).

163. Lang, E.K.: The accuracy of roentgenographic techniques in the diagnosis of renal mass lesions. Radiology (in prnit).

164. Lang, E.K.: Tumors arising within renal cysts. J Urol (in print).

165. Lang, E.K.: Staging of hypernephroma on basis of arteriography. J Urol (in print).

166. Lang, E.K.: Parapelvic cyst. (Diagnosis by arteriography and cyst puncture with double contrast study). Radiology (in print).

167. Laskownicki, A.: On diagnostic difficulties and possibilities of error in pararenal tumors. Pol Przegl Chir 35:Suppl:403-410, 1963 (Pol).

168. Lassen, H.K.: Geriatric practice, geriatric problems in surgery. A clinical review with a statistical survey of mortality rates as related to age. J Geront 17:167-179, 1962.

169. Lee, H.C., and Kay, S.: Hemangiopericytoma: Report of a case involving the kidney with an 11-year follow-up. Ann Surg 156:125-128, 1962.

170. Leger, L., and Levi, J.P.: Giant cancer of the kidney in cystic form. J Chir (Par) 79:50-62, 1960 (Fr).

171. Levine, S.R., Emmett, J.L., and Woolner, L.B.: Cyst and tumor occurring in the same kidney. J Urol 91:8-9, 1964.

172. Levine, S.R., Witten, D.M., and Greene, L.F.: Nephrotomography in Lindau Von Hippel's disease. J Urol 93:660-662, 1965.

173. Lhez, A., Caissel, J., and Leguevague, E.: Sur huit observations de kystes du rein. J Urol Nephrol (Paris) 71:645-647, 1965.

174. Liberthal, F.: Perirenal and peripelvic fibrolipomatosis: Their relationship to replacement lipomatosis of kidney. Surg Gynec and Obst 61:794-801, 1935.

175. Lillard, R.L., Keyting, W.S., and Daywitt, A.L.: 4-phase nephrotomo-

graphy in the diagnosis of renal cysts and tumors. Am J Roentgenal 99:593-599, 1967.

176. Lindblom, K.: Percutaneous puncture of renal cysts and tumors. Acta Radiol 27:66-72, 1946.

177. Lindblom, K.: Diagnostic kidney puncture of cysts and tumors. Amer J Roentgenol 68:209-215, 1952.

178. Ljunggren, E.: Partial nephrectomy in renal tumour. Acta Chir Scand (Suppl) 253:37-44, 1960.

179. Lombardo, S.: Acute anemia caused by perirenal hematoma in angiomyolipoma of the kidney. Minerva Chir 16:1181-1186, 1961. (It)

180. Lopatkin, N.A.: Diagnosis and treatment of solitary serous cysts of the kidney. Urologiia 29:12-17, 1964. (Rus)

181. Lopez Engelking, R., Alpuche Morales, E., and Maldonaldo, M.D.: Adenocarcinoma mucinoso primario de la pelvis renal. Rev Mex Urol 23:301-307, 1964.

182. Loutfi, A.H., and Abd-El-Haleem, S.: Lymphangioma of the kidney. J Egypt Med Assoc 42:622-626, 1959.

183. Love, L., and Frank, S.J.: Angiographic features of angiomyolipoma of the kidney. Amer J Roentgenol 95:406-408, 1965.

184. McDonald, J.R., and Priestley, J.T.: Malignant tumors of the kidney; Surgical and prognostic significance of tumor thrombosis of the renal veins. Surg Gynec Obst 77:295-306, 1943.

185. McGowan, A.J., Jr., and Ippolito, J.J.: Infected solitary renal cyst. J Urol 93:559-561, 1965.

186. McIntyre, H.: Diagnostic percutaneous renal puncture. J Canad Assoc Radiol 15:126-130, 1964.

187. McKenzie, K.R.: Xanthogranulomatous pyelonephritis: Confusion with renal carcinoma. J Urol 92:261-262, 1964.

188. McQueeney, A.J., Dahlen, G.A., and Gebhart, W.F.: Cystic hamartoma (Angiomyolipoma) of kidney simulating renal carcinoma. J Urol 92:98-102, 1964.

189. Malament, M.: The diagnosis of renal cyst versus renal carcinoma. Surg Clin N Amer 45:1377-1392, 1965.

190. Mann, L.T.: Spontaneous disappearance of pulmonary metastases after nephrectomy for hypernephroma: 4-year follow-up. J Urol 59:564-569, 1948.

191. Marsico, G., Rocca, P., and Giorgi, G.: Differential angiographical aspects of renal cysts and tumors. Ann Radiol Diagn (Bologna) 36:160-178, 1963. (It)

192. Masset, A., and Balo, J.: Multiple kidney adenomas. Maly Onkol 7:81-86, 1963. (Hun)

193. Meaney, T.F., and Stewart, B.H.: Selective renal angiography: An integral part of the management of renal mass lesions. J Urol 96:644-650, 1966.

194. Meissner, H.: Uber adenomatose Neubildungen der Niere. Urol Int 16: 228-240, 1963.

195. Melicow, M.M., and Gile, H.H.: A hypernephroma in a polycystic kidney: Review of literature and report of a case. J Urol 43:767-773, 1940.

196. Mertz, J.H.O., Lang, E.K., and Klingerman, J.J.: Percutaneous renal biopsy utilizing cine fluoroscopic monitoring. J Urol 95:618-621, 1966.

197. Miller, H.C.: Use of C-reactive protein in distinguishing renal cyst from tumor. Inves Urol 1:514-517, 1964.

198. Minami, T., Chino, I., Ishibash, A., et al: Parapelvic cyst. Acta Urol Jap 11:750-756, 1965. (Jap)

199. Montella, G., Nahni Costa, P., and Turba, E.: Il cistadenoma papillifero del rene. Arch Ital Urol 36:237-274, 1963 (5 ref).

200. Montero, J.: Quistes renales asociados a carcinoma. Arch Esp Urol 17: 246-250, 1964.

201. Morin, L.J., and Albert, D.J.: Milk of calcium stone in renal cyst. J Urol 96:869-870, 1966.

202. Morris, J.G., Corey, G.J., Dick, R., Evans, W.A., Smitanando, N., Pearson, B.S., Loewenthal, J.I., Blackburn, C.R.B., and McRae, J.: The diagnosis of renal tumors by radioisotope scanning. J Urol 97:40-54, 1967.

203. Mostofi, F.K.: "Pathology and spread of renal carcinoma" in King, J.S. (ed) Renal neoplasia. Boston, Little, Brown and Co, 1967, pp. 45-85.

204. Musacchio, F., and Mitchell, N.: Primary renal echinococcosis: A case report. Amer J Trop Med 15:168-171, 1966.

205. Myers, G.H., Jr., Fehrenbaker, L.G., and Kelalis, P.P.: Prognostic significance of renal vein invasion by hypernephroma. J Urol 100: 420-423, 1968.

206. Nakamura, M., and Isobe, Y.: Solitary cyst and pelvic papilloma occurring in the same kidney: report of a case. Acta Urol Jap 8:292-298, 1962. (Jap)

207. Narciso, F.V., Jr., and Basa, G.F.: Renal angiolipoleimyoma. Case report and histogentic concepts. Philipp J Cancer 4:210-214, 1962.

208. Nersisian, R.K.: Parapelvic cyst of the kidney. Urologiia 28:50-51, 1963. (Rus)

209. Ng, E., Rossiter, S.B., and Reimer, G.W.: Renal puncture. A neglected aid in the diagnosis of renal masses. Calif Med 104:102-105, 1966.

210. Nicoloff, D.M.: Renal arteriovenous fistula: Occurrence in renal cell carcinoma. Amer J Surg 108:82-84, 1964.

211. Ochsner, M.G.: Renal cell carcinoma: Five-year follow-up study of 70 cases. J Urol 93:361-363, 1965.

212. Olsson, O.: Roentgen examination of the kidney and the ureter: in

Handbuch der Urologie; Diagnostic Radiology, Springer, Berlin, 1962.

213. Parker, R.M., Timothy, R.P., and Harrison, J.H.: Neoplasia of solitary kidney. J Urol 101:283-286, 1969.

214. Patel, J., Cormier, J.M., and Artur, E.: L'Angiomyolipome renal, cause Possible d'hematome perinephretique trop negemment dit "spontane". Mem Acad Chir (Paris) 91:769-772, 1965.

215. Pearlman, C.K.: Coexisting renal carcinoma and Cyst. J Int Coll Surg 41:620-631, 1964.

216. Pearman, R.O.: Percutaneous needle puncture and aspiration of renal cysts: A diagnostic and therapeutic procedure. J Urol 96:139-145, 1966.

217. Pennisi, S.A., Russi, S., and Bunts, R.C.: Multiple dissimilar tumors in one kidney. J Urol 78:205-211, 1957.

218. Petersen, C.C., Jr., Jackson, J.H., Jr., and Moore, J.G.: Reevaluation of nephrotomography stressing limitations of the procedure. J Urol 98:721-727, 1967.

219. Petkovic, S.D.: An anatomical classification of renal tumors in the adult as a basis for prognosis. J Urol 81:618-623, 1959.

220. Petraroia, F., Jannell, O., and Sorrentino, R.: Le cisti solitarie del rene (contributo clinico-statistico). Acta Med Ital, Med Trop 19:41-50, 1964.

221. Phillips, D.E.: The percutaneous aspiration of renal cysts. Proc Roy Soc Med 56:928-930, 1963.

222. Phillips, T.L., Chin, F.G., and Palubiuskas, A.J.: Calcifications in renal masses: an 11-year survey. Radiology 80: 786-794, 1963.

223. Plaine, L.I., and Hinman, F., Jr.: Malignancy in asymptomatic renal masses. J Urol 94:342-347, 1965.

224. Potampa, P.B., and Schneider, I.J.: Bilateral true primary papillary carcinoma of the kidneys. J Urol 86:522-524, 1961.

225. Price, E.B., Jr., and Mostofi, F.K.: Symptomatic angiomyolipoma of the kidney. Cancer 18:761-774, 1965.

226. Quenu, L.: Rhabdomyosarcoma of the right kidney. J Urol Nephrol (Paris) 69:263-266, 1963. (Fr)

227. Rabinowitz, J.G., Wolfe, B.S., and Goldman, R.H.: Roentgen features of renal adenomas. Radiology 84:263-269, 1965.

228. Ranniger, K.: Selective renal arteriographic appearance of necrotic hypernephroma. Radiology 83:414-418, 1964.

229. Ravich, L., Lerman, P.H., and Bates, S.: Two primary clear cell carcinomas in the same kidney: a case report. J Urol 92:267-269, 1964.

230. Rehm, R.A., Taylor, W.N., and Taylor, J.N.: Renal cyst associated with carcinoma. J Urol 86:307-309, 1961.

231. Reisner, K., and van de Weyer, K.H.: Nephrotomography: Technic, indications and limitations. Rontgenblatter 21:9-15, 1969. (Ger)

232. Reiss, M.: Traumatic rupture of renal cortical cyst into the calyceal system. Am J Roentgenol 101:696-699, 1967.

233. Riches, E.W., Griffith, I.H., and Thackray, A.C.: New growths of the kidney and ureter. Brit J Urol 23:297-356, 1951.

234. Rieser, C., and Deitch, M.J.: Value of renal angiography in everyday urologic practice. J Urol 96:24-30, 1966.

235. Rigoli, E., and Manetti, E.: Le cisti pielogeniche. Inquadramento patogenetico e relazioni con le malformazioni cistiche della niedollare renale. Riv Anat Pat Oncol 24:1331-1347, 1963.

236. Robson, C.J.: Radical nephrectomy for renal cell carcinoma. J Urol 89:37-42, 1963.

237. Robson, C.J., Churchill, B.M., and Anderson, W.: Results of radical nephrectomy for renal cell carcinoma. J Urol 101:297-301, 1969.

238. Rognon, L.M., Guntz, M., and Simard, C.: Cancer renal evoquant un kyste calcifie. J Urol Nephrol (Paris) 71:618-623, 1965.

239. Roijer, A.: Angiographische Diagnostick eines kleinen Nierentumors. Radiologe 3:426-427, 1963.

240. Rosenthall, L.: Radionuclide diagnosis of malignant tumors of the kidney. Am J Roentgenol 101:662-668, 1967.

241. Rouffilange, F.: Tumor of the kidney with a simple cystic form. J Urol Nephrol. (Paris) 68:431-433, 1962. (Fr)

242. Rubin, R.: Comment: National cooperative study. JAMA 204:232-233, 1968.

243. Salik, J.O., and Abeshouse, B.S.: Calcifications and cartilage formation in the kidney. Am J Roentgenol 88:125-143, 1962.

244. Sankaran, V.: Fibrosarcoma of the kidney. J Ind St Med Assoc 43:81-83, 1964.

245. Sato, S., Takano, M., and Chiba, E.: Fibroma of the kidney with cyst. Report of a case and review of the literature. Acta Med Biol (Niigata) 11:99-104, 1963.

246. Schapiro, A., Wellington, P., and Gonick, H.: Urinary beta-glucuronidase in urologic diseases of the kidney. J Urol 100:146-157, 1968.

247. Schencker, B., Marcure, R.W., and Moody, D.L.: Simplified nephrotomography. A drip infusion technique. Amer J Roentgenol 95:283-289, 1965.

248. Schreiber, M.H., and Rea, V.E.: The resectability of carcinoma of the kidney. Am J Roentgenol 104:343-349, 1968.

249. Scholl, A.J.: Peripelvic cysts of kidney: Report of 2 cases. JAMA 136:4-7, 1948.

250. Seshanarayana, K.N., and Keats, T.E.: Angiomyolipoma of the kidney. Am J Roentgenol 104:332-334, 1968.

251. Shapiro, R.: Peripelvic renal cyst. Case report with a diagnostic roentgen sign. Amer J Roentgenol 90:81-82, 1963.

252. Shockman, A.T.: The significance of ring-shaped renal calcifications. J Urol 101:438-442, 1969.

253. Shucksmith, H.S.: Fibroma of the renal pelvis. Brit J Urol 35:261-262, 1963.

254. Simpson, W.: Curvilinear calcification in renal carcinomata. Brit J Urol 38:129-132, 1966.

255. Small, M.P., Anderson, E.E., and Atwill, William, H.: Simultaneous bilateral renal cell carcinoma: Case report and review of the literature. J Urol. 100:8-14, 1968.

256. Smith, M.J.V., Nanson, E.M., and Campbell, J.H.: An unusual case of closed rupture of the ureter. J Urol 83:277-278, 1960.

257. Southwood, W.F., and Marshall, V.F.: A clinical evaluation of nephrotomography. Brit J Urol 30:127-141, 1958.

258. Stackpole, R.H.: Treatment of carcinoma in a solitary kidney. Case report and review of the literature. J Urol 93:353-360, 1965.

259. Sukthomya, C., and Levin, B.: Pseudotumors of kidney secondary to anticoagulant therapy. Radiology 88:701-703, 1967.

260. Swynegedauw, J., Rozan, R., and Giaux, G.: Les criteres de fonctionnment renal d'apres le nephrogramme a l'hippuran. J Radiol Electr 46:358-362, 1965.

261. Thackray, A.C.: "Pathology and spread of renal adenocarcinoma" in tumors of the kidney and ureter. E. W. Riches (ed), London: E and S Livingstone Ltd, 1964, pp. 72-86.

262. Thompson, G.J., and Culp, O.S.: Perplexing cystic masses near the kidney. J Urol 89:370-376, 1963.

263. Thurn, P., and Bucheler, E.: Die Nephrotomographie. Fortschr Roentgenstr 99:784-794, 1963.

264. Tovena, A.: Malignant renal cystadenoma. Minerva Med 50:3009-3015, 1959. (It).

265. Trabucco, A.E., Saubidet, J.A., and Bruno, P.: Cripto-tumor renal. Rev Argent Urol 32:164-167, 1963.

266. Truc, E., Grasset, D., Badosa, J., Balmes, M., Dossa, J., and Cormier, M.: Voluminous calcified cystic tumor of the kidney. J Urol Nephrol (Paris) 68:804-806, 1962. (Fr)

267. Uchuguna, A.F.: Intraparenchymatous solitary cyst of the kidney. Urologiia 29:51-52, 1964. (Rus)

268. Uson, A.C., and Melicow, M.M.: Multilocular cysts of kidney with intrapelvic herniation of a "daughter" cyst: Report of 4 cases. J Urol 89:341-348, 1963.

269. Uson, A.C., Melicow, M.M., and Lattimer, J.K.: Is renal arteriography (aortography) a reliable test in the differential diagnosis between kidney cysts and neoplasms? J Urol 89: 554-559, 1963.

270. Uson, A.C., Melicow, M.D., and Schwarz, G.S.: Hydronephrosis due to aberrant blood vessels versus communicating peripelvic cysts: Their roentgenographic diagnosis. Amer J Roentgen 90:109-114, 1963.

271. Vasko, J.S., Broc-man, S.K., and Bomar, R.L.: Renal angiomyolipoma: A rare cause of spontaneous massive retroperitoneal hemorrhage. Ann Surg 161:577-581, 1965.

272. Viamonte, M., Jr., Ravel, R., Politano, V., and Bridges, B.: Arteriographic findings in patient with tuberous sclerosis. Am J Roentgenol 98:723-733, 1966.

273. Vinik, M., Freed, T.A., Smellie, W.A.B., Chir, M., and Weidner, W.: Xanthogranulomatous pyelonephritis: Angiographic considerations. Radiology 92:537-540, 1969.

274. Walsh, A.: Solitary cyst of the kidney and its relationship to renal tumour. Brit J Urol 23:377-379, 1951.

275. Watkins, K.H.: Cysts of kidney due to hydrocalycosis. Brit J. Urol 11: 207-215, 1939.

276. Watson, R.C., Fleming, R.J., and Evans, J.A.: Arteriography in diagnosis of renal carcinoma: Review of 100 cases. Radiology 91:888-897, 1968.

277. Wellauer, J.: Solitary kidney cyst with hematuria. Fortschr Roentgenstr 95:137-138, 1961. (Ger)

278. Weyeneth, R.: L'Indication du reno-vasogramme en urologie, son importance dans le diagnostic — differentiel entre cancer et kyste solitaire du rein. Bibl Gastroent 8:206-227, 1965.

279. Weyrauch, H.M., and Fleming, A.E.: Congenital hydrocalycosis: Hydrocalycosis of single renal calyx in newborn infant with complete destruction of kidney. J Urol 63:582-587, 1950.

280. Wheeler, B.C.: Use of aspirating needle in diagnosis of solitary renal cysts. New Engl J Med 226:55-57, 1942.

281. Whitmore, E.R.: Hypernephroid tumors of the kidney. South Med J 29:1051-1062, 1936.

282. Williams, G., Blandy, J.D., and Tressida, G.C.: Communicating cysts and diverticula of the renal pelvis. Brit J Urol 61:163-170, 1969.

283. Windholz, F.: Roentgen appearance of central fat tissue of kidney: Its significance in urography. Radiology 56:202-213, 1951.

284. Winkel, K. zum, Keiser, D. von, Muller, H., et al: Szintigraphie und angiographie der Nieren. Strahlentherapie 128:43-55, 1965.

285. Wise, M.F.: Differentiation between renal cyst and carcinoma. J Urol 101:137-139, 1969.

286. Witherington, R., and Rinker, J.R.: Percutaneous needle puncture in the diagnosis of renal cysts. J Urol 95:733-737, 1966.

287. Witten, D.M., Greene, L.F., and Emmett, J.L.: An evaluation of nephrotomography in urologic diagnosis. Am J Roentgenol 90:115-123, 1963.

288. Wrobel, S.: Apropos of the diagnosis of solitary cysts. Pol Przegl Chir 36:Suppl:1303-1308, 1964. (Pol)

289. Yekel, R.L., and Tesluk, H.: Angiomyolipoma of the kidney. Bull Mayo Clin 15:93-100, 1961.

290. Zak, F.G.: Self-healing hypernephromas. J Mt Sinai Hosp 24:1352-1356, 1957.

AUTHOR INDEX

171

SUBJECT INDEX